Craniofacial Trauma

Editor

DEBORAH R. SHATZKES

NEUROIMAGING CLINICS OF NORTH AMERICA

www.neuroimaging.theclinics.com

Consulting Editor
SURESH K. MUKHERJI

August 2014 • Volume 24 • Number 3

ELSEVIER

1600 John F. Kennedy Boulevard • Suite 1800 • Philadelphia, Pennsylvania, 19103-2899

http://www.neuroimaging.theclinics.com

NEUROIMAGING CLINICS OF NORTH AMERICA Volume 24, Number 3
August 2014 ISSN 1052-5149, ISBN 13: 978-0-323-32018-4

Editor: John Vassallo (j.vassallo@elsevier.com)
Developmental Editor: Donald Mumford

Neuroimaging Clinics of North America (ISSN 1052-5149) is published quarterly by Elsevier Inc., 360 Park Avenue South, New York, NY 10010-1710. Months of issue are February, May, August, and November. Business and editorial offices: 1600 John F. Kennedy Blvd., Suite 1800, Philadelphia, PA 19103-2899. Business and editorial offices: 6277 Sea Harbor Drive, Orlando, FL 32887-4800. Periodicals postage paid at New York, NY, and additional mailing offices. Subscription prices are USD 360 per year for US individuals, USD 514 per year for US institutions, USD 180 per year for US students and residents, USD 415 per year for Canadian individuals, USD 655 per year for Canadian institutions, USD 525 per year for international individuals, USD 655 per year for international institutions and USD 260 per year for Canadian and foreign students and residents. To receive student/resident rate, orders must be accompanied by name of affiliated institution, date of term, and the *signature* of program/residency coordinator on institution letterhead. Orders will be billed at individual rate until proof of status is received. Foreign air speed delivery is included in all *Clinics* subscription prices. All prices are subject to change without notice. POSTMASTER: Send address changes to *Neuroimaging Clinics of North America*, Elsevier Health Sciences Division, Subscription Customer Service, 3251 Riverport Lane, Maryland Heights, MO 63043. Telephone: 1-800-654-2452 (U.S. and Canada); 314-447-8871 (outside U.S. and Canada). Fax: 314-447-8029. E-mail: journalscustomerservice-usa@elsevier.com (for print support); journalsonlinesupport-usa@elsevier.com (for online support).

Reprints. For copies of 100 or more of articles in this publication, please contact the Commercial Reprints Department, Elsevier Inc., 360 Park Avenue South, New York, NY 10010-1710. Tel.: 212-633-3874; Fax: 212-633-3820; E-mail: reprints@elsevier.com.

Neuroimaging Clinics of North America is covered by *Excerpta Medical/EMBASE,* the RSNA Index of Imaging Literature, *MEDLINE/PubMed (Index Medicus),* MEDLINE/MEDLARS, SciSearch, Research Alert, and Neuroscience Citation Index.

PROGRAM OBJECTIVE

The goal of *Neuroimaging Clinics of North America* is to keep practicing radiologists and radiology residents up to date with current clinical practice in radiology by providing timely articles reviewing the state of the art in patient care.

TARGET AUDIENCE

Practicing radiologists, radiology residents, and other healthcare professionals who utilize neuroimaging findings to provide patient care.

LEARNING OBJECTIVES

Upon completion of this activity, participants will be able to:

1. Review surgical perspectives in craniofacial trauma.
2. Discuss skull base fractures and associated complications.
3. Recognize considerations in pediatric craniofacial trauma.

ACCREDITATION

The Elsevier Office of Continuing Medical Education (EOCME) is accredited by the Accreditation Council for Continuing Medical Education (ACCME) to provide continuing medical education for physicians.

The EOCME designates this enduring material for a maximum of 15 *AMA PRA Category 1 Credit*(s)™. Physicians should claim only the credit commensurate with the extent of their participation in the activity.

All other health care professionals requesting continuing education credit for this enduring material will be issued a certificate of participation.

DISCLOSURE OF CONFLICTS OF INTEREST

The EOCME assesses conflict of interest with its instructors, faculty, planners, and other individuals who are in a position to control the content of CME activities. All relevant conflicts of interest that are identified are thoroughly vetted by EOCME for fair balance, scientific objectivity, and patient care recommendations. EOCME is committed to providing its learners with CME activities that promote improvements or quality in healthcare and not a specific proprietary business or a commercial interest.

The planning committee, staff, authors and editors listed below have identified no financial relationships or relationships to products or devices they or their spouse/life partner have with commercial interest related to the content of this CME activity:

Gregory D. Avey, MD; Dane M. Barrett, MD; Kristen L. Baugnon, MD; J. Levi Chazen, MD; J. Jared Christophel, MD; Alisa D. Gean, MD; Lindell R. Gentry, MD; Ajay Gupta, MD; Kristen Helm; Patricia A. Hudgins, MD, FACR; Brynne Hunter; Mohannad Ibrahim, MD; Tabassum A. Kennedy, MD; Bernadette L. Koch, MD; Joshua Lantos, MD; Sandy Lavery; Carlos Leiva-Salinas, MD; Gary G. Lelli, Jr, MD; Jill McNair; Sugoto Mukherjee, MD; Suresh K. Mukherji, MD, MBA, FACR; Sara R. Nace, MD; C. Douglas Phillips, MD, FACR; Paul J. Schmitt, MD; Mark E. Shaffrey, MD; Deborah R. Shatzkes, MD; Karthikeyan Subramaniam; Alina Uzelac, DO; John Vassallo.

The planning committee, staff, authors and editors listed below have identified financial relationships or relationships to products or devices they or their spouse/life partner have with commercial interest related to the content of this CME activity:

Hemant A. Parmar, MD has a research grant from Siemens Corporation.

UNAPPROVED/OFF-LABEL USE DISCLOSURE

The EOCME requires CME faculty to disclose to the participants:

1. When products or procedures being discussed are off-label, unlabelled, experimental, and/or investigational (not US Food and Drug Administration (FDA) approved); and
2. Any limitations on the information presented, such as data that are preliminary or that represent ongoing research, interim analyses, and/or unsupported opinions. Faculty may discuss information about pharmaceutical agents that is outside of FDA-approved labelling. This information is intended solely for CME and is not intended to promote off-label use of these medications. If you have any questions, contact the medical affairs department of the manufacturer for the most recent prescribing information.

TO ENROLL

To enroll in the *Neuroimaging Clinics of North America* Continuing Medical Education program, call customer service at 1-800-654-2452 or sign up online at http://www.theclinics.com/home/cme. The CME program is available to subscribers for an additional annual fee of $235 USD.

METHOD OF PARTICIPATION

In order to claim credit, participants must complete the following:

1. Complete enrolment as indicated above.
2. Read the activity.
3. Complete the CME Test and Evaluation. Participants must achieve a score of 70% on the test. All CME Tests and Evaluations must be completed online.

CME INQUIRIES/SPECIAL NEEDS

For all CME inquiries or special needs, please contact elsevierCME@elsevier.com.

NEUROIMAGING CLINICS OF NORTH AMERICA

Contributors

CONSULTING EDITOR

SURESH K. MUKHERJI, MD, MBA, FACR
Professor and Chairman; W.F. Patenge
Endowed Chair, Department of Radiology,
Michigan State University, East Lansing,
Michigan

EDITOR

DEBORAH R. SHATZKES, MD
Professor of Radiology, Hofstra North Shore -
LIJ School of Medicine; Director of Head and
Neck Radiology, Lenox Hill Hospital and The
New York Head and Neck Institute, North
Shore LIJ Health System, New York, New York

AUTHORS

GREGORY D. AVEY, MD
Assistant Professor, Department of Radiology,
Clinical Science Center, University of
Wisconsin-Madison, Madison, Wisconsin

DANE M. BARRETT, MD
Resident Physician, Department of
Otolaryngology-Head and Neck Surgery,
University of Virginia Health System,
Charlottesville, Virginia

KRISTEN L. BAUGNON, MD
Assistant Professor of Radiology, Department
of Radiology and Imaging Sciences, Emory
University School of Medicine, Atlanta, Georgia

J. LEVI CHAZEN, MD
Assistant Professor, Department of Radiology,
Weill Cornell Medical College, New York,
New York

J. JARED CHRISTOPHEL, MD
Division of Head and Neck Surgical Oncology;
Assistant Professor, Division of Facial Plastic &
Reconstructive Surgery, Department of
Otolaryngology-Head and Neck Surgery,
University of Virginia Health System,
Charlottesville, Virginia

ALISA D. GEAN, MD
Clinical Professor of Neuroradiology; Adjunct
Professor of Neurology and Neurosurgery,
Department of Radiology, Brain and Spinal
Injury Center (BASIC), San Francisco
General Hospital, University of California,
San Francisco, San Francisco, California

LINDELL R. GENTRY, MD
Professor, Department of Radiology,
Clinical Science Center, University of
Wisconsin-Madison, Madison, Wisconsin

AJAY GUPTA, MD
Assistant Professor, Department of Radiology,
Weill Cornell Medical College, New York,
New York

PATRICIA A. HUDGINS, MD
Professor of Radiology, Department of
Radiology and Imaging Sciences, Emory
University School of Medicine, Atlanta,
Georgia

MOHANNAD IBRAHIM, MD
Associate Professor, Department of Radiology,
University of Michigan Health System,
Ann Arbor, Michigan

TABASSUM A. KENNEDY, MD
Assistant Professor, Department of Radiology,
Clinical Science Center, University of
Wisconsin-Madison, Madison,
Wisconsin

BERNADETTE L. KOCH, MD
Associate Director Radiology, Department of
Radiology, Cincinnati Children's Hospital
Medical Center; Professor of Radiology and
Pediatrics, University of Cincinnati College of
Medicine, Cincinnati, Ohio

JOSHUA LANTOS, MD
Radiology Resident, Department of Radiology,
Weill Cornell Medical College, New York,
New York

CARLOS LEIVA-SALINAS, MD
Fellow Physician, Division of Neuroradiology,
Department of Radiology and Medical Imaging,
University of Virginia Health System,
Charlottesville, Virginia

GARY J. LELLI Jr, MD
Assistant Professor, Department of
Ophthalmology, Weill Cornell Medical College,
New York, New York

SUGOTO MUKHERJEE, MD
Assistant Professor, Division of Neuroradiology,
Department of Radiology and Medical Imaging,
University of Virginia Health System,
Charlottesville, Virginia

SURESH K. MUKHERJI, MD, MBA, FACR
Professor and Chairman; W.F. Patenge
Endowed Chair, Department of Radiology,
Michigan State University, East Lansing,
Michigan

SARA R. NACE, MD
Neuroradiology Fellow/Clinical Instructor,
Department of Radiology, University of
Wisconsin-Madison, Madison, Wisconsin

HEMANT A. PARMAR, MD
Associate Professor, Department of Radiology,
University of Michigan Health System,
Ann Arbor, Michigan

C. DOUGLAS PHILLIPS, MD, FACR
Professor, Department of Radiology, Weill
Cornell Medical College, New York, New York

PAUL J. SCHMITT, MD
Resident Physician, Department of
Neurological Surgery, University of Virginia
Health System, Charlottesville, Virginia

MARK E. SHAFFREY, MD
David D. Weaver Professor and Chairman,
Department of Neurological Surgery, University
of Virginia Health System, Charlottesville,
Virginia

ALINA UZELAC, DO
Assistant Clinical Professor of Neuroradiology,
Department of Radiology, San Francisco
General Hospital, University of California,
San Francisco, San Francisco, California

Contents

> Over the last two decades, there has been a marked increase in the number of computed tomography (CT) studies performed in the United States, with a resultant increase in the radiation dose delivered to patients. Hence there is an urgent need to optimize CT protocols and to get familiar with the factors affecting the CT radiation dose and with available dose reduction options. This article discusses the basic physics related to CT technique and describes current and future methods of dose reduction. Also briefly described are other CT techniques applicable in the maxillofacial region, such as three-dimensional CT, cone beam CT, and dual-energy CT.

> This article reviews the importance of particular radiologic findings related to facial trauma and their implications for clinical and surgical management. An emphasis is placed on critical imaging signs that warrant immediate surgical attention.

> In the clinical assessment of orbital trauma, visual acuity and extraocular muscle motility are critical for rapid evaluation of injury severity. However, assessment of these parameters may be limited by edema and concomitant injuries. Imaging may further delineate the trauma pattern and extent of injury. This review focuses on orbital soft-tissue injuries that can exist with or without orbital fracture. Imaging techniques and soft-tissue injuries, including those involving the anterior chamber, iris and ciliary body, lens, globe, posterior segment, and optic nerve, are reviewed, in addition to intraocular foreign bodies and cavernous-carotid fistulas.

> Basilar skull fractures are a relatively frequent occurrence in significant head trauma, and their detection is important, as even linear nondisplaced fractures can be associated with critical complications. The management of skull base fractures depends on the location and extent of these associated complications. This article reviews skull base anatomy; morphology of the common fracture patterns within the anterior,

central, and posterior skull base; associated complications; imaging findings; and possible pitfalls in imaging of skull base trauma.

Imaging of Temporal Bone Trauma   467

Tabassum A. Kennedy, Gregory D. Avey, and Lindell R. Gentry

Temporal bone trauma is commonly seen in patients with craniofacial injury and can be detected using multidetector computed tomography. A thorough understanding of the different types of temporal bone fracture patterns is needed to accurately describe the trajectory of injury as well as anticipated complications. Fractures should be described based on direction, segment of temporal bone involved, as well as involvement of the otic capsule. More importantly, the radiologist plays an integral role in identifying complications of temporal bone injury, which often have significant clinical implications.

Cerebrovascular Trauma   487

Sara R. Nace and Lindell R. Gentry

Significant progress has been made recently in the recognition, screening, diagnosis, and treatment of blunt cerebrovascular vascular injury (BCVI). Although controversy still exists as to optimal screening algorithms and best diagnostic modality, the vital and growing role of noninvasive imaging in identifying patients at high risk for BCVI and in characterizing the injury itself has been clearly established. There has been promising early work in stratifying BCVI patients into risk categories by initially evaluating them with high-resolution head, maxillofacial, and cervical computed tomographic examinations with the ultimate goal of maximizing diagnostic yield and enabling prompt initiation of therapy.

Pediatric Considerations in Craniofacial Trauma   513

Bernadette L. Koch

In many respects, craniofacial trauma in children is akin to that in adults. The appearance of fractures and associated injuries is frequently similar. However, the frequencies of different types of fractures and patterns of injury in younger children vary depending on the age of the child. In addition, there are unique aspects that must be considered when imaging the posttraumatic pediatric face. Some of these are based on normal growth and development of the skull base and craniofacial structures, and others on the varying etiologies and mechanisms of craniofacial injury in children, such as injuries related to toppled furniture, nonaccidental trauma, all-terrain vehicle accidents, and impalement injuries.

Surgical Perspectives in Craniofacial Trauma   531

Paul J. Schmitt, Dane M. Barrett, J. Jared Christophel, Carlos Leiva-Salinas, Sugoto Mukherjee, and Mark E. Shaffrey

Knowledge of relevant anatomy and underlying mechanisms of traumatic injury is essential for understanding the radiologic findings in craniofacial trauma and their clinical importance. Craniofacial anatomy is diverse, and as a result of this anatomic diversity, physicians from numerous different specialties scrutinize similar imaging sets, looking for different pathologic abnormalities within the same anatomic regions. Radiologists familiar with the chief concerns of this anatomically diverse region can help expedite the decision-making process by keeping those concerns in mind when they report their findings. This review provides an overview of situations wherein surgical management may be indicated.

Foreword
Craniofacial Trauma

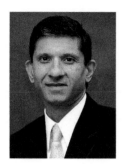

Suresh K. Mukherji, MD, MBA, FACR
Consulting Editor

It is my distinct pleasure to have Dr Deborah Shatzkes as our Editor for this issue of *Neuroimaging Clinics*. It gives me great pride to be able to call Deborah a close friend and colleague for nearly 20 years. She is a gifted educator, excellent researcher, and dedicated leader in Head and Neck Radiology. Her practice is 100% Head and Neck Radiology, and therefore, she has tremendous experience and case material.

This issue is focused on craniofacial trauma, which is one of Deborah's many areas of expertise. This issue is a timely and practical topic that will be pertinent to anyone who interprets cases from the emergency room. The issue begins with an article on optimizing CT technique followed by articles on orbital and facial fractures, soft tissue injuries, skull base trauma, and cerebrovascular injuries. There is an article dedicated to pediatric craniofacial trauma that focuses on the unique aspects of pediatric trauma compared with adult trauma. This issue is further enhanced by the inclusion of an ophthalmologist to provide important clinical context to this material.

I sincerely thank Dr Shatzkes for this important contribution, which will be an instant "classic." More importantly, I also want to thank Deborah for being such a wonderful friend, colleague, and confidant throughout my professional career.

Suresh K. Mukherji, MD, MBA, FACR
Professor and Chairman
W.F. Patenge Endowed Chair
Department of Radiology
Michigan State University
846 Service Road
East Lansing, MI 48824, USA

E-mail address:
mukherji@rad.msu.edu

Neuroimag Clin N Am 24 (2014) xi
http://dx.doi.org/10.1016/j.nic.2014.06.002
1052-5149/14/$ – see front matter © 2014 Published by Elsevier Inc.

Preface
Craniofacial Trauma

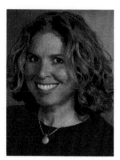

Deborah R. Shatzkes, MD
Editor

Anyone who works anywhere near an emergency department will inevitably encounter craniofacial trauma, whether from the perspective of a clinician or an imager. Findings of facial trauma may be visible on only the lowest images of a head CT, or the highest images of a cervical spine CT, but they nonetheless must be noted and attended to. In this issue of *Neuroimaging Clinics*, we attempt to explore the spectrum of imaging findings in craniofacial trauma, with particular emphasis on what is most important for the clinicians to know. With this in mind, we hope this issue will be of value to neuroradiologists, general radiologists, and surgeons.

We begin with an article on optimizing CT technique, a discussion of particular relevance in today's era of public concern with radiation exposure. Cutting-edge techniques aimed at reducing exposure while optimizing resolution are presented in a pragmatic fashion that will facilitate publication to practice utilization. Next, a comprehensive article on orbital and facial fractures is followed by another article on associated soft tissue injuries. The inclusion of an ophthalmologist among the authors ensures that the review of ocular trauma, an area with which radiologists tend to be less familiar, is accurate, relevant, and complete.

The article on skull base trauma and its complications focuses on the prevalent and clinically important problem of CSF leak, presenting both classic and emerging imaging techniques and accompanied by a thorough review of skull base anatomy. Moving to the lateral skull base, we focus next on temporal bone trauma, where fracture classification is emphasized, along with imaging findings that may herald associated complications. We next move to a comprehensive review of the related issue of cerebrovascular trauma, acknowledging that identification of vascular injuries is always a clinical priority. As we know, children are not just small adults, and a treatment of the specific imaging findings and clinical issues in pediatric craniofacial trauma follows. Finally, we synthesize all we have learned in an article written by surgeons and focusing specifically on what radiologists must include in their reports to be of real value to the multidisciplinary teams that manage these complicated patients.

It was an honor and true pleasure to coordinate this issue, which includes contributions from established experts and rising stars in the field. I appreciate all their efforts immensely. I'd like to thank Dr Suresh Mukherji for inviting me to guest edit this issue. The team at Elsevier has been unfailingly professional and incredibly helpful throughout this process. Finally, I'd like to thank my husband, Doug Phillips, who has been my official and nonofficial partner in numerous editing efforts, including this one.

Deborah R. Shatzkes, MD
Hofstra North Shore - LIJ School of Medicine
Lenox Hill Hospital and
The New York Head and Neck Institute
North Shore LIJ Health System
New York, NY 10075, USA

E-mail address:
Shatzkes@hotmail.com

neuroimaging.theclinics.com

Optimizing Craniofacial CT Technique

 CrossMark

Hemant A. Parmar, MD[a,*], Mohannad Ibrahim, MD[a], Suresh K. Mukherji, MD, MBA[b]

KEYWORDS

- Maxillofacial • CT • Technique • Optimization

KEY POINTS

- Over the last decade there has been escalating concern regarding the increasing radiation exposure stemming from CT examinations.
- It is becoming increasingly important to optimize CT imaging protocols and to apply dose-reduction techniques to ensure optimal imaging with the lowest possible dose.
- Several other advancements of CT technique applicable to the craniofacial region including three-dimensional CT, cone beam CT, and dual-energy CT are now widely used to best possible information about various craniofacial pathologies.

INTRODUCTION

Technological advances in computed tomography (CT) have generated a dramatic increase in the number of CT studies, with resultant increase in the radiation dose to patients. CT accounts for less than 20% of medical imaging studies, but approximately 60% of diagnostic imaging radiation dose.[1] Newer developments and usage of ultrasound and magnetic resonance imaging have failed to substantially reduce the overall number of CT examinations. In many instances, the CT scan is the first and only diagnostic imaging examination performed. In addition, advent of helical multidetector CT techniques with rapid acquisition times and newer applications, such as CT angiography, perfusion CT, and dual-energy CT, have led to a further increase in CT examinations. The overall increase in radiation dose is causing increasing concern among the radiologic community and general public alike.

The US Food and Drug Administration has established guidelines to address the growing concern over CT-associated radiation dose.[2] Their recommendations center on optimizing CT protocols and encouraging elimination of inappropriate CT referrals and unnecessary repeat examinations. The basic pillars of dose reduction include justification of the study and eliminating inappropriate CT referrals, limiting scan range to the region of interest, limiting the number of contrast phases, and use of a relatively large pitch (**Box 1**). The goal is a radiation dose as low as reasonably achievable. Radiation dose delivered to the patient is proportional to the amount of energy delivered by the photons within the x-ray beam. This depends on the number of the photons and the individual photon energy, which is dictated by the image acquisition parameters, such as kilovoltage (kilovolt [peak]), tube current (milliampere), and x-ray tube rotation time along with such other factors as slice thickness, scan coverage, and pitch. Additionally, body habitus and size of the patient are important factors for the radiation dose delivered, especially for pediatric patients and small adults. There have been several

[a] Department of Radiology, University of Michigan Health System, 1500 East Medical Center Drive, Ann Arbor, MI 48109, USA; [b] Department of Radiology, Michigan State University, 846 Service Road, East Lansing, MI 48824, USA

* Corresponding author. Department of Radiology, University of Michigan, Taubman Center/B1/132 F, 1500 East Medical Center Drive, Ann Arbor, MI 48105.

E-mail addresses: hparmar@umich.edu; parurad@hotmail.com

Neuroimag Clin N Am 24 (2014) 395–405
http://dx.doi.org/10.1016/j.nic.2014.03.004

neuroimaging.theclinics.com

Box 1
Pillars of CT dose reduction

- Justification of the CT study/elimination of inappropriate CT referrals
- Limiting CT scan range to the region of interest
- Limiting the number of contrast phases
- Use of a relatively large pitch
- Use of automated tube current modulation
- Use of adaptive dose shielding
- Use of newer image reconstruction algorithms

Box 2
Maxillofacial CT parameters for adults

Scan type	Helical
HiRes mode	On
Gantry rot time/length	0.5 s full
Detector coverage	20 mm
Slice thickness	0.625 mm
Interval	0.625 mm
Pitch	0.969:1
Speed	19.37
kVp	100
mA	250
ASIR %	30
% of dose reduction	None
Recon mode	Plus
SFOV	Head
DFOV	16–18
Algorithm	HD Bone Plus
WW/WL	4000/1000

Generate axial, coronal, and sagittal reformats in both standard and bone algorithm

DFOV	Optimize
Thickness	2.5 mm
Spacing	2.5 mm
Render mode	Average
WW/WL (bone)	4000/1000
WW/WL (standard)	350/50

advances in dose reduction techniques. These include tube current modulation, peak voltage optimization, noise reduction reconstruction algorithms, adaptive dose collimation, and improved detection system efficiency. It is imperative for practicing radiologists to be familiar with these dose reduction techniques and to optimize the imaging protocols to get the best possible images with the least possible dose.

This article discusses the basic physics related to CT technique and describes current and future methods of dose reduction. Also briefly described are other CT techniques applicable in the maxillofacial region, such as three-dimensional CT, cone beam CT (CBCT), and dual-energy CT. We provide CT scanning parameters used at our institutions for the maxillofacial region in adults and children (**Boxes 2** and **3**).

CT RADIATION DOSE MEASUREMENT

CT scans involve continuous exposure around the patient by the rotating gantry in the region to be examined. This leads to almost uniform deposition of energy with a relatively symmetric gradient from the surface toward the center of the patient. Because of x-ray scattering, deposition of the radiation beam energy often extends beyond the directly scanned volume into the adjacent tissues. Therefore, the radiation dose in the scanned section is the summation of the dose because of the direct beam in the scanned plane and dose contributions from radiation scattering in the adjacent tissues. The conventional metric representing the integrated dose of the direct irradiation of the scanned volume and the scattered radiation from the adjacent scanned volumes is the computed tomography dose index (CTDI) measured in milligrays (10^{-3} Gy).[3] CTDI is defined as the dose profile of a single x-ray tube rotation integrated

Box 3
Maxillofacial CT parameters for children

Scan type	Helical
HiRes mode	On
Gantry rot time/lengths	0.5 s full
Detector coverage	20 mm
Slice thickness	0.625 mm
Interval	0.625 mm
Pitch	0.531
Speed	10.62
kVp	100
mA 0–3 years	80
mA 3–12 years	100
mA 12+ years	120
ASIR %	30
% of dose reduction	None
Recon mode	Plus
SFOV	Ped head
SFOV 12+ years	Small head
DFOV	Optmize
Algorithm	HD Bone Plus
WW/WL	4000/1000

Generate axial, coronal, and sagittal reformats in both standard and bone algorithm

DFOV	Optimize
Thickness	2 mm
Spacing	2 mm
Render mode	Average
WW/WL (HD bone)	4000/1000
WW/WL (HD standard)	350/50

over a scan length in the z-direction, and normalized to the table travel per tube rotation in a scan with pitch 1. The CTDI is equivalent to the multiple scan average dose, which is the average dose in the center region of the scan range over which a CT scan is performed.[3] The $CTDI_{vol}$ is defined as $CTDI_w$/pitch. The value of $CTDI_{vol}$ multiplied by the length of the scan (in centimeters) is known as the dose-length product (DLP) and is usually measured in units of milligray-centimeters (mGy-cm). The DLP is commonly reported on the CT scanner for each CT study and is included in the patient dose report. When considering the potential dose from the CT scan, the metric to take into consideration is the DLP because it contains the CTDI that is a measure of scanner output for a particular scanning technique and the total scanning length along the patient's body.

CT ACQUISITION PARAMETERS
Beam Energy

The energy of the incident x-ray beam is determined by the kilovolt (peak). Any variation in tube potential causes substantial change in CT radiation dose. When all other parameters are held constant and the kilovolt (peak) is decreased, the radiation dose also decreases. The relationship between the change in effective dose and tube potential is exponential.[4] In general, lower kilovolt (peak) yields better contrast especially for bone and iodine (Fig. 1), with the effect being much smaller for soft tissues, such as fat and muscle.[5] Lowering the kilovolt (peak) settings and increasing the milliamperes, either by using automatic tube current modulation or using a technique chart, is considered one of the most effective strategies to reduce radiation dose while maintaining image quality.[6,7] Moreover, lowering the kilovolt (peak) increases vascular enhancement because the attenuation of iodine-based contrast agents increases with reduced photon energy distribution because of the high atomic number of iodine[8] and the effect of the iodine k-edge in the x-ray attenuation at such energy levels (Fig. 2).

Photon Fluence

The photon fluence, determined by the milliampere and gantry rotation time (seconds), has a direct effect on patient radiation dose. The radiation dose is directly proportional to the milliampere value, with the radiation dose increasing linearly with increasing milliamperes. Any decrease in tube current should be considered carefully, because such reduction causes an increase in image noise, which may affect the diagnostic outcome of the examination.[9]

Collimation, Table Speed, and Pitch

The helical (or spiral) acquisition has introduced new acquisition parameters, such as table speed and pitch, which is defined as the ratio of table feed per gantry rotation to the nominal beam width. The pitch value has a direct influence and is inversely proportional to the patient radiation dose (Dose ~1/pitch).[10,11] The effect of pitch on radiation dose and image quality is negated in scanners that use an "effective milliampere

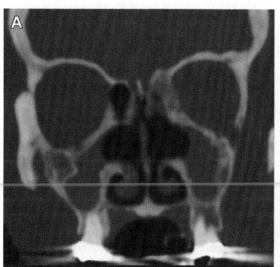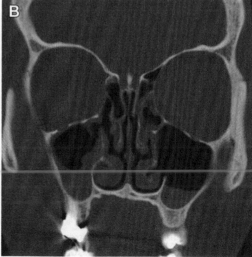

Fig. 1. Different kilovolt (peak) and milliampere settings for bone. Coronal CT of maxillofacial bones performed in two different patients. (*A*) First patient was scanned at 250 mA and 140 kVp. (*B*) Second patient was scanned at 150 mA and 100 kVp resulting in significantly better quality image with more than 50% reduction of DLP.

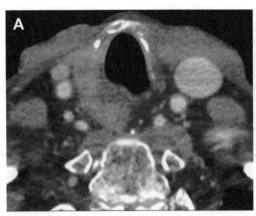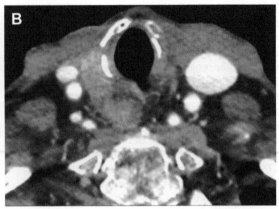

Fig. 2. Different kilovolt (peak) setting for iodine. (*A*) Axial CT of the neck in a patient scanned at 140 kVp compared with (*B*) axial CT image of the neck in same patient scanned with 100 kVp. There is improved contrast and increased attenuation of the blood vessels with lower kilovolt (peak) technique.

setting" (defined as milliampere divided by pitch).[12] In such scanners, constant effective milliampere value is held irrespective of pitch value, by adjusting the tube current and adjusting the tube current-time product approximately proportional to the changes in pitch. This keeps the radiation dose relatively constant despite variation of pitch. Moreover, an increase in the pitch value in modern scanners equipped with automatic milliampere modulation (discussed later) does not necessarily lead to dose reduction because the milliampere is automatically adjusted to account for the increase in the pitch.

CURRENT STRATEGIES IN DOSE REDUCTION
Automated Tube Current Modulation

Automated tube current modulation (ATCM), also known as automatic exposure control, is one of the most widely available technical innovations for significant radiation dose reduction. ATCM allows constant image quality in the CT examination at a lower radiation dose regardless of the patient's body habitus or the attenuation characteristics of the body part being scanned. It can be preprogrammed or may adjust by using a feedback circuit based on the attenuation value of the preceding image, or a combination of the two. ATCM allows automatic adjustment of the tube current in the x, y plane (angular modulation), along the z-axis (longitudinal modulation), or both (combined modulation) to maintain a user-selected noise level in the image.[13] Longitudinal modulation adjusts the tube current along the z-axis, which results in a lower tube current in the neck region with higher tube current at the skull base and shoulder level, rendering the images of similar noise. Angular modulation adjusts the

tube current within the same slice, with increased tube current in the lateral projection compared with the anteroposterior projection.

Adaptive Dose Shielding

Helical CT imaging acquires additional data with several extra gantry rotations before the beginning and after the end of the scanned volume, a process called overranging (or z overscanning). The extra data are needed for the interpolation required in the image reconstruction of a helical acquisition of the scanned volume. The adaptive dose shield is a technology based on precise and independent movement of collimator blades that limit this overranging. The collimator asymmetrically opens at the beginning and closes at the end of each spiral scan, blocking the parts of the x-ray beam that are not used for image reconstruction. The proportion of radiation dose reduction depends on the scan range, detector collimation, and pitch, and has been shown to range from 7% to 38%.[14,15]

Image Reconstruction Algorithms

Iterative reconstruction (IR) algorithm was the first algorithm applied to generate CT images from raw data. It was computationally demanding and resulted in long reconstruction time. IR accurately models the data collection process in CT by generating a set of synthesized projections and incorporating details of the scanner's geometric information, such as focal spot size, detector cell size, and the shape and size of each image voxel.[16] IR was replaced by filtered back projection (FBP) technique, which is an analytical reconstruction technique that operates on several fundamental assumptions about the scanner geometry and offers a compromise between reconstruction speed and image noise. A major drawback for FBP algorithm is increased image noise that stems from the fact that FBR assumes noiseless projection data, which then must be overpowered by increasing the radiation dose. With improvement in computational power, IR is once again being considered for noise suppression and artifact reduction with lowering the radiation dose. Major CT manufacturers are implementing their own IR methods to achieve dose reduction without image-quality degradation. These include Adaptive Statistical Iterative Reconstruction (ASIR) algorithm and more recently a model-based IR technique (VEO) from GE Healthcare System (Milwaukee, WI), Iterative Reconstruction in Image Space and Sinogram-Affirmed Iterative Reconstruction from Siemens (Enlargen, Germany), Adaptive Iterative Dose Reduction from Toshiba Medical Systems (Tokyo, Japan),[17,18] and iDose from Philips Healthcare (Best, Netherlands).

ASIR is a recently introduced reconstruction algorithm for CT that uses statistical models to reduce noise.[19] In ASIR, information obtained from an FBP algorithm is used as an initial building block for image reconstruction. The ASIR model then uses matrix algebra to estimate the value of adjacent pixels. This is repeated over numerous iterations and the actual value of a pixel is compared with the estimated pixel value that the model predicts. By comparing these values, the model is then able to selectively identify and subtract noise from the image.[20] Such advances have led to the logical hypothesis that the reduced noise and thus potentially improved image quality achieved with ASIR could be leveraged to reduce radiation dose while preserving overall image quality (**Fig. 3**). ASIR images may appear to have an unusual "texture" particularly when the radiation dose used is not sufficiently low. In clinical practice, using variable blending levels of image reconstruction with FBP and ASIR techniques can be performed to generate clinically acceptable images.

FUTURE ADVANCEMENT IN DOSE REDUCTION
Automated Organ-based Current Modulation

This technique reduces the tube current for certain projections to avoid direct exposure to radiosensitive organs, such as the thyroid gland and ocular lens.[17] It modulates the current along the z-axis according to the body habitus. In the x- and y-planes the current is decreased over the 120-degree radial arc, whereas it is increased in the remaining 240-degree arc. The dose in the prescribed projection can be near zero, which capitalizes on the fact that only 180 degrees of data plus the fan angle are necessary to reconstruct a CT image.[17]

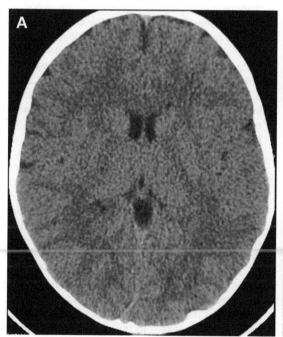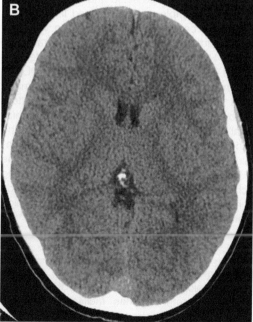

Fig. 3. ASIR for pediatric head CT. Axial CT images in two different 3-year-old patients at the level of basal ganglia. (*A*) Without ASIR technique. (*B*) With ASIR technique. No qualitative differences in image quality are appreciated.

Automated (Optimized) Tube Voltage Modulation

Conventional dose modulation techniques modulate the tube current, whereas the tube voltage (the kilovolt [peak] setting) is left unchanged. However, there is a large potential for dose reduction by optimizing the tube kilovolt (peak) setting. Such optimization of the kilovolt (peak) setting can be performed automatically for each individual patient and specific examination by analyzing the information gathered by the topogram (scout view) to optimize kilovolt (peak) and milliampere to maintain a certain contrast-to-noise ratio. This improves the selection of kilovolt (peak) for a particular examination beyond manual kilovolt (peak) selection.

Noise Reduction Algorithm with Image Reconstruction and Data Processing

Improving the overall image quality with lower noise levels can be achieved using optimally designed data processing and image reconstruction methods without sacrificing other image properties. Computational advancement has allowed the use of sophisticated reconstruction methods to control noise and streak artifact in the projection data domain before image reconstruction. As CT manufacturers present different IR methods to achieve lower noise, newer versions of such methods are being introduced allowing for further reduction of CT image noise and hence radiation dose. For example, a model-based IR algorithm (VEO) has been introduced following ASIR to achieve further noise reduction and lower radiation dose.[20] Hoxworth and colleagues[21] have demonstrated sinus CT using Veo with a mean DLP of 37.4 mGy-cm and significantly reduced image noise in comparison with FBP, and resultant improved image quality for evaluation of craniofacial soft tissue structures. Unfortunately, the smoothing effect of the Veo model-based IR impairs evaluation of such structures as thin bone at a low dose.[21] Several image-based filtering techniques usually perform quite well with regards to reducing image noise while maintaining high contrast resolution.[17]

Three-dimensional Reconstruction

Three-dimensional CT has become an essential tool in craniofacial surgery. Advent of helical CT and multidetector CT has facilitated scanning by dramatically reducing data acquisition time. Three-dimensional CT is useful not only for preoperative assessment and surgical simulation but also for postoperative evaluation. Its ability to generate three-dimensional surface images and two-dimensional images in any desired plane (multiplanar reconstruction) permits analysis of morphologic changes of the craniofacial skeleton and its surrounding soft tissues with much more precision than any previously available modalities (Fig. 4). It permits focus on specific areas of clinical and surgical concern, such as visualizing bone fragments from all angles and planes. In addition to the extent of fracture, the potential mechanism of the injury may be readily assessed. This is true for craniofacial injuries because these injuries often produce marked edema not only limiting clinical examination but additionally producing haziness on conventional radiographs that may obscure underlying bony injuries.[22] Thin structures (the base of the skull, the orbital floor, the hard palate) and the floor of the mouth may be adequately evaluated with multiplanar reconstructions.[22] Moreover, three-dimensional CT reformation is extremely useful for patient and family consultation and education.

CBCT

Conventionally, dental and maxillofacial imaging has mainly relied on panoramic and intraoral radiography; however, these two-dimensional modalities provide insufficient information and produce superimposition of anatomic structures that can impair visualization of complex anatomy during diagnosis and treatment planning. Although standard CT scanners with three-dimensional dataset can be used for maxillofacial and dental applications, their radiation doses are quite high.[23] Because of low radiation dose and accurate three-dimensional imaging, a dental CT scanner based on CBCT is become increasingly popular in diagnosis and treatment planning for dental and maxillofacial applications (Fig. 5).[24,25] CBCT uses X rays much more efficiently, requires far less electrical energy, and allows for the use of smaller and less expensive x-ray components than fan-beam technology. As expected, CBCT offers lower radiation dose compared with standard CT machines: the integral absorbed radiation dose of radiation was less than one-fifteenth that of spiral CT when the exposure condition of the latter was optimized.[24] The CBCT machine cost is less expensive than standard CT machines and the machine size is smaller, allowing it to be easily installed in physicians' clinics. Additionally, isotropic CT scans reconstructed with CBCT make it unnecessary to reposition the patient for direct coronal imaging. Sagittal images are also feasible with these isotropic data. This is extremely useful to eliminate metallic streak artifacts from

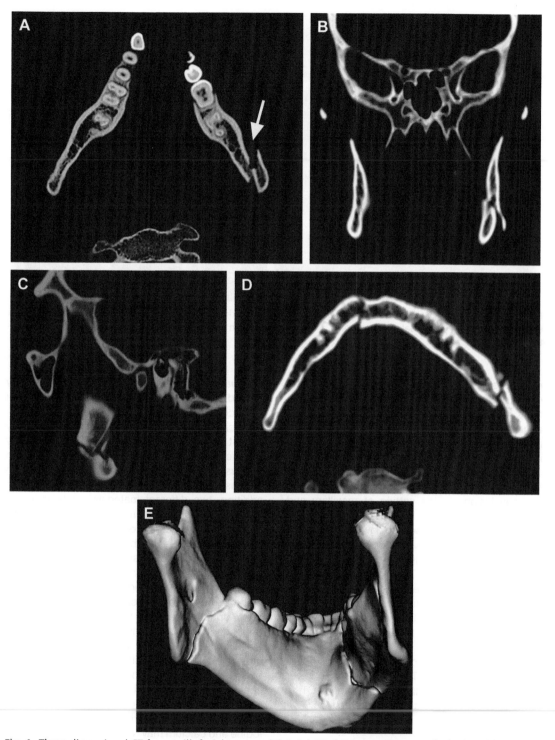

Fig. 4. Three-dimensional CT for maxillofacial trauma. (*A*) Axial CT of the mandible reveals displaced fracture of the left mandible (*arrow*). Coronal (*B*) and sagittal (*C*) reformatted images depict the same fracture. The patient also had another fracture on right side. (*D*) Curved reformatted image, performed to image the whole mandible, nicely depicts both fractures on one single image. (*E*) Three-dimensional reconstructed image of the mandible, viewed from posteriorly, shows both fractures.

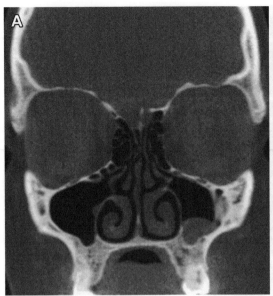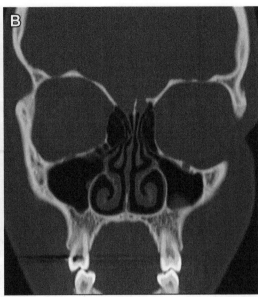

Fig. 5. Cone beam CT. Maxillofacial CT in a patient obtained with cone beam CT (*A*) and regular multidetector CT (*B*). Depiction of paranasal sinus anatomy and sinus disease on cone beam CT is comparable with multidetector CT.

radiodense dental hardware and in eliminating the need for special patient positioning. Several authors[26–28] have demonstrated excellent image acquisition for different structures, such as morphology of the mandible, location of the inferior alveolar canal, and even for the relationship of radiopaque templates to the bone. It should be noted that CBCT was designed to scan osseous lesions in the setting of maxillary and mandibular diseases. It is incapable of discriminating soft tissue because of its low contrast resolution and, if soft tissue evaluation is needed, either conventional CT or magnetic resonance imaging should be considered.

Recently, CBCT has been shown to produce images of sufficient resolution to diagnose fractures of the orbital floor and to show impingement of the rectus muscle in the fracture line. Retrobulbar hemorrhage, however, was not identified on CBCT because of poor contrast sensitivity. The radiation dose from CBCT was significantly lower than the lowest dose from conventional CT in terms of effective dose and dose to the lens.[29]

Dual-energy CT

The concept of multienergy CT has been known from the beginning of the CT era.[30] However, it is only recently that technical advancements made it possible to construct devices capable of generating two x-ray beams of low and high energy within a short time span. On conventional CT, the attenuation of materials in each voxel is directly related to the ratio of the linear x-ray attenuation coefficient of the material to the linear attenuation coefficient of water at the effective x-ray energy in that voxel.[31] Single-energy CT numbers may not accurately represent material composition because the effective energy varies with location because of x-ray beam hardening and scatter. In addition, two different materials, such as iodine and calcium, with different elemental composition could have the same Hounsfield unit (HU) measurement because of their similar linear attenuation coefficients despite differing in mass attenuation coefficient and material density. With dual-energy CT, two image datasets are acquired in the same anatomic location using two different x-ray spectra to allow the analysis of energy-dependent changes in the attenuation of different tissues.[30] Each type of tissue material demonstrates a relatively specific change in attenuation between images obtained with a high-energy spectrum and those obtained with a low-energy spectrum. This attenuation difference allows better characterization of the tissue. For example, iodine and calcium may demonstrate similar attenuation on conventional CT images; however, the attenuation of iodine increases markedly more than calcium on dual-energy CT images obtained with low energy versus images obtained with high energy.[32] At present, three types of dual-energy CT scanners are available that differ in the technique used to acquire high- and low-energy CT datasets: (1) a dual-source dual-energy scanner, (2) a single-source dual-energy scanner with fast kilovolt (peak) switching (ie, rapid alternation between high and low kilovolt [peak] settings), and (3) a single-source dual-energy scanner with dual detector layers.

Gemstone spectral imaging (GSI) is a type of dual-energy CT technology that acquires images with fast switching and acquisition of two separate energy levels (80 and 140 kVp). GSI creates a spectral HU curve that displays the attenuation in HU units of any tissue across the 40- to 140-keV range. Although the linear attenuation coefficient of substances decreases with increasing kiloelectron volt, different materials show different rates of

decline, and this principle is exploited to enhance the contrast between two different tissues at any selected kiloelectron volt.[33] Another advantage of GSI CT is its ability to calculate the effective atomic number Z ("effective Z") of any voxel by measuring the liner coefficient at two different tube potentials, which can help identify different tissue types. Recent studies have demonstrated that spectral HU curves derived from dual-energy GSI CT is a promising technique for the differentiation of benign and malignant neck pathologic findings (**Fig. 6**A-D).[34] Although the exact reason why malignant tissues display significant increases in HU over benign tissues at lower virtual kiloelectron volt is unknown, it may be caused by

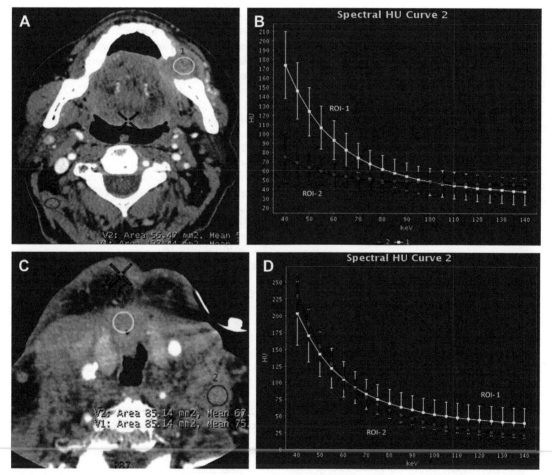

Fig. 6. Dual-energy CT. (*A*) Contrast-enhanced axial CT image in a 65-year-old man with biopsy-proved squamous cell cancer of left mandible. Region of interest (ROI) is placed in the lesion (1) and right paraspinal muscle (2). (*B*) Spectral Hounsfield unit (HU) curves of the same regions as *A* are depicted. Curve 1 is derived from the left mandibular mass and curve 2 from the normal paraspinal muscle. There is difference in the HU scale for two ROI with much higher HU range in the malignant lesion. (*C*) Contrast-enhanced axial CT image in a 76-year-old man with previous laryngeal cancer and now presenting with benign posttreatment change. ROI are placed within this lesion and left paraspinal muscle. (*D*) Spectral HU curves show no significant differences between the two ROIs suggesting benign nature of the laryngeal lesion. (*Courtesy of* Ashok Srinivasan, MD, Ann Arbor, MI.)

neoangiogenesis and/or higher capillary permeability in malignancies that permit relatively increased contrast leakage (and hence iodine concentration).[35,36] With respect to trauma, dual-energy CT has been shown to provide significantly improved images in the presence of metal artifacts by using metal suppression techniques.[37] Dual-energy CT has also been shown to diagnose bone marrow edema in vertebral compression fractures on noncalcium images with a high specificity and a high positive predictive value when compared with magnetic resonance imaging.[38]

SUMMARY

There are significant variations between different sites and CT scanners in imaging protocols with resultant wide ranges of radiation dose for similar clinical indications. Furthermore, adult scan protocols have been directly applied to pediatrics without making proper adjustment for small patient size. Consequently, there is an urgent need to optimize CT protocols and to get familiar with the factors affecting the CT radiation dose and with available dose reduction options as discussed. Other advancements of CT technique applicable to the craniofacial region including three-dimensional CT, CBCT, and dual-energy CT have made it possible to acquire the best possible information on CT without compromising on radiation dose delivered to the patient.

REFERENCES

1. Zacharia TT, Kanekar SG, Nyugen DT, et al. Optimization of patient dose and image quality with z- axis dose modulation for computed tomography (CT) head in acute head trauma and stroke. Emerg Radiol 2011;18(103):107.
2. Feigal DW Jr. FDA public health notification: reducing radiation risk from computed tomography for pediatric and small adult patients. Int J Trauma Nurs 2002;8:1–2.
3. Bauhs JA, Vrieze TJ, Primak AN, et al. CT dosimetry: comparison of measurement techniques and devices. Radiographics 2008;28:245–53.
4. Schindera ST, Nelson RC, Yoshizumi T, et al. Effect of automatic tube current modulation on radiation dose and image quality for low tube voltage multidetector row CT angiography: phantom study. Acad Radiol 2009;16:997–1002.
5. Huda W, Scalzetti EM, Levin G. Technique factors and image quality as functions of patient weight at abdominal CT. Radiology 2000;217:430–5.
6. Mulkens TH, Marchal P, Daineffe S, et al. Comparison of low-dose with standard-dose multidetector

7. Waaijer A, Prokop M, Velthuis BK, et al. Circle of Willis at CT angiography: dose reduction and image quality—reducing tube voltage and increasing tube current settings. Radiology 2007;242:832–9.
8. Matsuoka S, Hunsaker AR, Gill RR, et al. Vascular enhancement and image quality of MDCT pulmonary angiography in 400 cases: comparison of standard and low kilovoltage settings. AJR Am J Roentgenol 2009;192:1651–6.
9. Kalra MK, Maher MM, Toth TL, et al. Strategies for CT radiation dose optimization. Radiology 2004; 230:619–28.
10. Primak AN, McCollough CH, Bruesewitz MR, et al. Relationship between noise, dose, and pitch in cardiac multi-detector row CT. Radiographics 2006;26: 1785–94.
11. McNitt-Gray MF, Cagnon CH, Solberg TD, et al. Radiation dose in spiral CT: the relative effects of collimation and pitch. Med Phys 1999;26:409–14.
12. Mahesh M, Scatarige JC, Cooper J, et al. Dose and pitch relationship for a particular multislice CT scanner. AJR Am J Roentgenol 2001;177:1273–5.
13. Lee CH, Goo JM, Ye HJ, et al. Radiation dose modulation techniques in the multidetector CT era: from basics to practice. Radiographics 2008;28:1451–9.
14. Tzedakis A, Damilakis J, Perisinakis K, et al. The effect of z overscanning on patient effective dose from multidetector helical computed tomography examinations. Med Phys 2005;32:1621–9.
15. Christner JA, Zavaletta VA, Eusemann CD, et al. Dose reduction in helical CT: dynamically adjustable z-axis x-ray beam collimation. AJR Am J Roentgenol 2010;194:W49–55.
16. Xu J, Mahesh M, Tsui BM. Is iterative reconstruction ready for MDCT? J Am Coll Radiol 2009;6:274–6.
17. Ibrahim M, Parmar HA, Mukherji SK. Raise the bar and lower the dose. Current and future strategies for radiation dose reduction in head and neck imaging. AJNR Am J Neuroradiol 2014;35(4): 619–24.
18. Thibault JB, Sauer KD, Bouman CA, et al. A three-dimensional statistical approach to improved image quality for multislice helical CT. Med Phys 2007;34: 4526–44.
19. Silva AC, Lawder HJ, Hara A, et al. Innovations in CT dose reduction strategy: application of the statistical iterative reconstruction algorithm. AJR Am J Roentgenol 2010;194:191–9.
20. Katsura M, Matsuda I, Akahane M, et al. Model-based iterative reconstruction technique for radiation dose reduction in chest CT: comparison with the adaptive statistical iterative reconstruction technique. Eur Radiol 2012;22:1613–23.
21. Hoxworth JM, Lal D, Fletcher GP, et al. Radiation dose reduction in paranasal sinus CT using
CT in cervical spine trauma. AJNR Am J Neuroradiol 2007;28:1444–50.

model-based iterative reconstruction. AJNR Am J Neuroradiol 2014;35(4):644–9.

22. Kaur J, Chopra R. Three dimensional CT reconstruction for the evaluation and surgical planning of mid face fractures: a 100 case study. J Maxillofac Oral Surg 2010;9:323–8.

23. Cavalcanti MG, Rocha SS, Vannier MW. Craniofacial measurements based on 3D-CT volume rendering: implications for clinical applications. Dentomaxillofac Radiol 2004;33:170–6.

24. Guerrero ME, Jacobs R, Loubele M, et al. State-of-the-art on cone beam CT imaging for preoperative planning of implant placement. Clin Oral Investig 2006;10:1–7.

25. van Steenberghe D, Naert I, Andersson M, et al. A custom template and definitive prosthesis allowing immediate implant loading in the maxilla: a clinical report. Int J Oral Maxillofac Implants 2002;17:663–70.

26. Hashimoto K, Arai Y, Iwai K, et al. A comparison of a new limited cone beam computed tomography machine for dental use with a multidetector row helical CT machine. Oral Surg Oral Med Oral Pathol Oral Radiol Endod 2003;95:371–7.

27. Ito K, Gomi Y, Sato S, et al. Clinical application of a new compact CT system to assess 3-D images for the preoperative treatment planning of implants in the posterior mandible. A case report. Clin Oral Implants Res 2001;12:539–42.

28. Nakagawa Y, Kobayashi K, Ishii H, et al. Preoperative application of limited cone beam computerized tomography as an assessment toll before minor oral surgery. Int J Oral Maxillofac Surg 2002;31:322–7.

29. Brisco J, Fuller K, Lee N, et al. Cone beam computed tomography for imaging orbital trauma—image quality and radiation dose compared with conventional multislice computed tomography. Br J Oral Maxillofac Surg 2014;52:76–80.

30. Alvarez RE, Macovski A. Energy-selective reconstruction in X-ray computerized tomography. Phys Med Biol 1976;21:733–44.

31. Hounsfield GN. Computerized transverse axial scanning (tomography). Description of system. Br J Radiol 1973;46:1016–22.

32. Kalender WA, Perman WH, Vetter JR, et al. Evaluation of a prototype dual-energy computed tomographic apparatus. I. Phantom studies. Med Phys 1986;13:334–9.

33. Watanabe Y. Derivation of linear attenuation coefficients from CT numbers for low-energy photons. Phys Med Biol 1999;44:2201–11.

34. Srinivasan A, Parker RA, Manjunathan A, et al. Differentiation of benign and malignant neck pathologies: preliminary experience using spectral computed tomography. J Comput Assist Tomogr 2013;37:666–72.

35. Ash L, Teknos TN, Gandhi D, et al. Head and neck squamous cell carcinoma: CT perfusion can help noninvasively predict intratumoral microvessel density. Radiology 2009;251:422–8.

36. Zima A, Carlos R, Gandhi D, et al. Can pretreatment CT perfusion predict response of advanced squamous cell carcinoma of the upper aerodigestive tract treated with induction chemotherapy? AJNR Am J Neuroradiol 2007;28:328–34.

37. Coupal TM, Mallinson PI, McLaughlin P, et al. Peering through the glare: using dual-energy CT to overcome the problem of metal artefacts in bone radiology. Skeletal Radiol 2014;43(5):567–75.

38. Wang CK, Tsai JM, Chuang MT, et al. Bone marrow edema in vertebral compression fractures: detection with dual-energy CT. Radiology 2013;269:525–33.

Orbital and Facial Fractures

Alina Uzelac, DO[a],*, Alisa D. Gean, MD[b]

KEYWORDS

- Facial buttresses • Nasofrontal outflow tract • Orbital blow-out • Orbital blow-in
- Naso-orbito-ethmoid fracture • Zygomaticomaxillary complex fracture
- Intermaxillary (maxillomandibular) fixation

KEY POINTS

- Knowledge of typical patterns of facial fractures is important because each pattern may be associated with its respective functional complications.
- Three-dimensional images are commonly used by surgeons for operative planning in restoration of alignment and correction of cosmetic deformities, but can be occasionally useful to the radiologist as a summary view of complex midface fractures.

INTRODUCTION

Traumatic facial fractures are caused most often by motor vehicle accidents, falls, and assaults.[1] At our level I trauma center, the interpretation of facial fractures is routine in daily imaging. By far the most common injuries are the fractures of the midface, followed by fractures of the lower face (mandible) and the upper face (frontal bone and superior orbital rim).[1] The partition of the face into thirds (upper, middle, and lower) has particular relevance for surgical intervention. This article reviews, from cranial to caudal, the most common fracture patterns and the clinical relevance of the imaging findings as they impact patient management.

Multidetector computerized tomography (CT) is the imaging study of choice currently used to evaluate acute and nonacute facial trauma. Axial submillimeter bone algorithm images with sagittal, coronal, and three-dimensional reformations are routinely obtained. Occasionally, such as in the detailed evaluation of the orbit, oblique reformations are useful. The three-dimensional images are particularly helpful for the assessment of complex facial deformities, preoperative planning, and patient consultation.

It is well known that traumatic collapse of the face has a "cushion" or "bumper" effect that helps dissipate the impact force and thereby protect the neurocranium and cervical spine. However, the distribution of forces via the areas of thicker bone (facial buttresses) may still be transmitted to the cranial vault and cervical spine. Awareness of the facial buttresses (**Figs. 1** and **2**) helps with the understanding of the fracture patterns and the identification of osseous segments that require surgical reconstruction for restoration of the normal facial skeleton.

FRONTAL SINUS

Fractures of the fronto-orbital bar (frontal boss, tuber frontalis) usually involve the outer table of the frontal bone and sinus (**Fig. 3**), but they may also involve both tables (**Fig. 4**). Extension of a frontal sinus fracture into the posterior sinus wall

Disclosures: None.
Funding Sources: None.
[a] Department of Radiology, San Francisco General Hospital, University of California, San Francisco, 1001 Potrero Avenue, 1X55, San Francisco, CA 94110, USA; [b] Department of Radiology, Brain and Spinal Injury Center (BASIC), San Francisco General Hospital, University of California, San Francisco, 1001 Potrero Avenue, 1X55, San Francisco, CA 94110, USA
* Corresponding author.
E-mail address: alina.uzelac@ucsf.edu

neuroimaging.theclinics.com

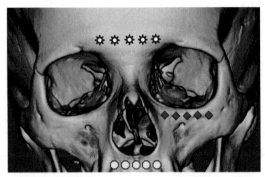

Fig. 1. Transverse midface buttresses: three-dimensional coronal reformatted CT demonstrates the three transverse buttresses of the midface: frontal (*white stars*), upper (*red diamonds*), and lower maxillary (*yellow circles*).

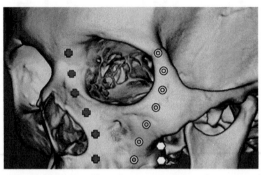

Fig. 2. Vertical midface buttresses: three-dimensional oblique reformatted CT demonstrates the three vertical buttresses of the midface: medial (*red crosses*), lateral (*white circles*), and posterior (pterygomaxillary, *yellow circles*).

results in communication with the anterior cranial fossa and may be associated with a dural tear and cerebrospinal fluid (CSF) leak. Potential intracranial spread of a pre-existing sinus infection may occur. In addition, these fractures are frequently associated with intracranial hemorrhage.

Isolated fractures of the inner table are uncommon and usually result from an occipital impact. Fractures through the medial aspect of the floor of frontal sinus typically involve the cribriform plate and fovea (roof) ethmoidalis and may result in a dural tear and/or chronic sinusitis. Fractures through the lateral aspect of the frontal sinus floor often involve the orbital roof (see Fig. 4A), depending on the lateral extent of frontal sinus pneumatization.

Frontal Sinus (Nasofrontal) Outflow Tract

Nasofrontal outflow tract injury is strongly suspected when the CT examination demonstrates involvement of the base of the frontal sinus, the anterior ethmoids, or both (Fig. 5). The posteromedial position of the nasofrontal outflow tract within the sinus makes it particularly susceptible to injury.[2]

Injury to the outflow tract can result in a frontal sinus mucocele and creation of an anaerobic environment with subsequent osteomyelitis and possible intracranial extension leading to a brain abscess. These complications may develop in delayed fashion, years after the inciting trauma.

Management of Frontal Sinus Fractures

A patent frontal sinus outflow tract deems the frontal sinus salvageable and the comminuted outer table is then repaired with plates and screws. If normal frontal sinus drainage pathway cannot be restored, the frontal sinus is surgically eradicated[3] by obliteration or cranialization (ie, the cranial cavity is expanded into the former sinus space). The nasofrontal outflow tract is eliminated with a graft. These procedures are best performed within 2 weeks posttrauma.

Frontal sinus obliteration is best achieved if, after the sinus mucosa is exenterated, the cavity is filled with vascularized pericranial flap (rather than devascularized abdominal fat, muscle, or bone graft).[4] The sinus mucosa is removed to

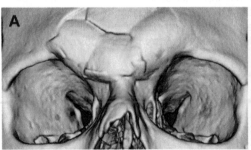

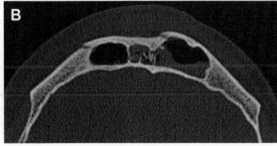

Fig. 3. Frontal orbital bar fracture with isolated involvement of the outer table of the frontal sinus. This 54-year-old male bicyclist went over the handle bars and landed on his forehead. (*A*) Coronal reformatted three-dimensional CT through the orbits demonstrates a comminuted, depressed fracture of the frontal bar. (*B*) Axial CT shows relative sparing of the inner table.

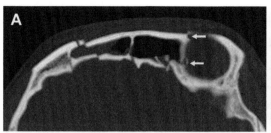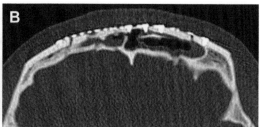

Fig. 4. Preoperative and postoperative views of a comminuted fracture involving both tables of the frontal sinus and orbital roof. (*A*) Preoperative axial CT shows the fracture extending into medial left orbital roof (*arrows*). (*B*) Postoperative CT demonstrates good cosmetic alignment following fixation of the outer table with mini-plates and screws.

prevent mucocele and subsequent mucopyocele formation.

Fractures that cause significant displacement of the posterior table and/or compromise of the dura are cranialized.[5] The posterior wall of the sinus is removed, the mucosa is meticulously stripped, and the dura and brain are brought to rest against the surgically repaired outer table of calvarium.

The management of frontal sinus fractures has become increasingly conservative because of the accumulated experience and the advent of endoscopic sinus surgery.[6] In the future, follow-up CT to ensure the absence of complications of conservatively managed fractures may likely be more frequently used.

Key points: frontal sinus fractures

1. Fracture through the frontal sinus base and/or anterior ethmoid implies possible involvement of nasofrontal outflow tract. If sinus patency cannot be restored, the sinus is sacrificed.

2. Involvement of frontal sinus posterior table increases the risk of CSF leak and intracranial infection.

ORBITAL TRAUMA
Blow-Out Orbital Fractures

An injury involving mainly the orbit is considered at higher risk of ocular trauma and optic nerve injury than orbital involvement by adjacent facial trauma. Isolated orbital fractures most commonly involve the weak medial orbital wall or floor, sparing the orbital rim, lead to enlargement of the orbit, and are known as blow-out fractures (**Fig. 6**). Enophthalmos can occur with large fragment blow-out fractures and its extent is best appreciated and repaired in delayed fashion, after the edema has resolved.

On CT evaluation, the presence of soft tissue herniation through the defect and the fracture size are important predictors of persistent diplopia. Somewhat surprisingly, small and medium size floor fractures with soft tissue herniation are more likely to cause entrapment than large floor fractures.[7] Any soft tissue incarceration at the fracture site may cause restriction as fibrous septa unite orbital tissue to the sheaths of the inferior rectus and oblique muscles making the diagnosis of entrapment a clinical one. Relatively large orbital floor fractures (**Fig. 7**) are at less risk for entrapment and, again, operative repair may be delayed.

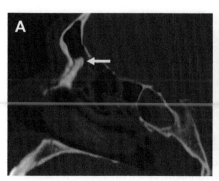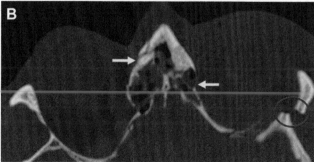

Fig. 5. Traumatic obstruction of the nasofrontal outflow tract. This 30-year-old man fell from a ladder onto his face. (*A*) Sagittal CT reformation shows a large nasoethmoidal fragment extending into the inferior frontal sinus (*arrow*) and obstructing the outflow tract. (*B*) Axial CT demonstrates bilateral comminution of the anterior ethmoids (*arrows*). A distracted fracture of the left superolateral orbital wall is also noted (*circle*).

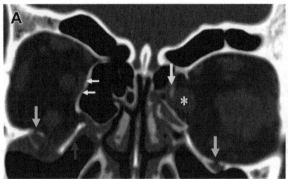
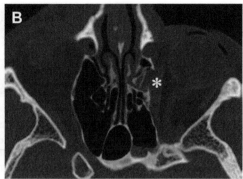

Fig. 6. Orbital blow-out fractures (inferior and medial). This 35-year-old man fell through a manhole. (A) Coronal and (B) axial CT images show bilateral orbital blow-out fractures: right orbital floor (*red arrow*) and left medial orbital wall (*yellow arrow*). The left medial rectus muscle (*yellow asterisk*) is enlarged, deformed, and medially displaced (*asterisk*). Compare with the normal right medial rectus extraocular muscle (*white arrows*). Note how the inferior blow-out fracture interrupts the inferior orbital foramen (*right blue arrow*), because all foramina are a point of weakness within the facial skeleton. Compare with the normal left inferior orbital foramen (*left blue arrow*).

Blow-In Orbital Fractures

The far less common blow-in fractures occur when the fractures fragments buckle within the orbit leading to a decrease in the orbital volume (Fig. 8). The decreased orbital volume, commonly aggravated by an intraorbital hematoma, leads to proptosis and poses risk of damage to the optic nerve.

Proptosis and Optic Nerve Injury

Orbital fractures are commonly accompanied by a subperiosteal intraorbital hematoma (Fig. 9) and less commonly associated with extensive orbital emphysema (Fig. 10), but both complications can result in proptosis. A large blow-out fracture results in actual decompression of the orbit and obviates the need for surgical hematoma evacuation. Severe proptosis with posterior globe tenting is an ophthalmologic emergency (Fig. 11).

Patients with fractures involving the optic canal (Fig. 12) require vigilant evaluation of the optic nerve because the edema and hematoma can rapidly result in vision loss. In most cases, traumatic optic neuropathy represents a nerve contusion caused by a blow to the superior orbital rim with the force transmitted to the optic canal.

The clinical challenge lies in the timely diagnosis of optic nerve injury to ensure rapid intervention. An afferent pupillary defect may be the only clinically reliable sign of traumatic optic neuropathy because many of these patients have suffered concomitant traumatic brain injury and routine ophthalmologic testing (ie, visual acuity, color vision, and visual field) cannot be easily performed.

Endoscopic surgical decompression is usually reserved for an obvious optic canal hematoma or bone fragment impinging on the nerve.[8] The International Optic Nerve Trauma Study concluded that

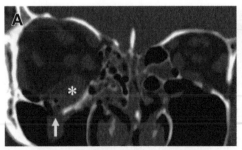
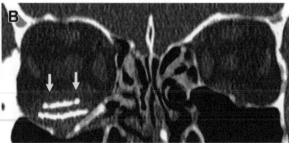

Fig. 7. Inferior orbital blow-out fracture. (A) Coronal reformation obtained immediately after the patient's fall from a ladder shows an inferior orbital extraconal hematoma (*asterisk*) inseparable from inferior rectus muscle. Note the subjacent depressed orbital floor fracture (*arrow*). (B) Coronal CT demonstrating reconstruction of the orbital floor that was performed 16 months postinjury because the patient developed enophthalmos and diplopia in all fields of gaze. An expected small postoperative hematoma (*arrows*) is seen surrounding the Medpor implant at 2 weeks.

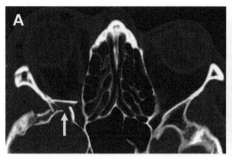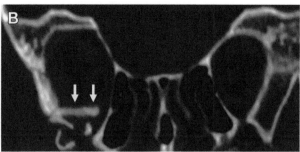

Fig. 8. Orbital blow-in fracture. (*A*) Axial CT image demonstrates a comminuted fracture of the right sphenotemporal buttress with a fracture fragment extending into the right orbital apex (*arrow*). (*B*) The coronal reformation shows the volume of the right orbit reduced by the fracture fragments that are protruding from below (*arrows*). Impingement of the inferior rectus muscle is also suspected.

decompression should be reserved for worsened or not improving visual acuity.[9] In addition, at our institution, the use of steroids for treatment of optic nerve trauma has been abandoned given the questionable benefit and the known morbidity associated with steroid administration.

Complications of Orbital Roof Fractures

Immediately posttrauma, intraorbital herniation of contused brain parenchyma may mimic a subperiosteal hematoma (**Fig. 13**). Follow-up imaging may reveal a traumatic meningoencephalocele that can be misinterpreted as an orbital neoplasm (**Fig. 14**).

Key points: orbital fractures

1. Proptosis resulting in posterior globe tenting is an ophthalmologic emergency.

2. Large fragment blow-out fractures can lead to enophthalmos after the edema subsides.

3. Smaller fragment orbital blow-out fractures are more likely to cause entrapment.

4. Clinical entrapment may occur even in the setting of normal extraocular muscle position and morphology on CT.

5. Fractures involving the optic canal imply a high risk for optic nerve injury. Fragments into the optic canal need to be emergently removed to salvage vision.

---

posttrauma. The remainder of patients usually responds to decrease of intracranial pressure by temporary use of a lumbar subarachnoid drain and only a small number require endoscopic placement of a graft at the site of CSF leak.[10]

If precise localization of a persistent CSF leak is desired, a CT cisternogram is performed. A baseline noncontrast sinus CT is obtained for purposes of comparison with images obtained following intrathecal contrast administration. Under intermittent lumbar imaging guidance, never more than 10 mL (given the risk of provoking a seizure) of Omnipaque-300 nonionic iodinated contrast is introduced into the thecal sac by lumbar puncture. The patient is then placed in a prone Trendelenburg position to facilitate intracranial flow of contrast. Even though a 25-minute wait is recommended, some patients may be scanned earlier, because arrival of the contrast within the intracranial subarachnoid space may be signaled by the development of a headache. Obtaining a delayed single image through the brain at the level of the sinuses objectively confirms the contrast opacification of subarachnoid space and a repeat CT of the sinuses in prone position is then performed.

Identification of the exact location of CSF leakage is important (**Fig. 15**). However, either an intermittent leak or rapid filling of nasal cavity or sinuses because of a large CSF fistula may hinder the diagnosis. In addition, blood products also have high density and their presence may obscure contrast extravasation.

CEREBROSPINAL FLUID LEAK

CSF rhinorrhea or orbitorrhea occurs in a small percentage of facial fractures and is most commonly encountered with nasoethmoid complex fractures. CSF is confirmed by detection of β2 transferrin in the fluid collected. Fortunately, most CSF leak cases spontaneously resolve within the first week

---

Cisternogram pitfalls

1. Intermittent CSF leakage.

2. Rapid leakage of contrast into nasal cavity or paranasal sinus.

3. Residual traumatic blood products in the sinuses or nasal cavity.

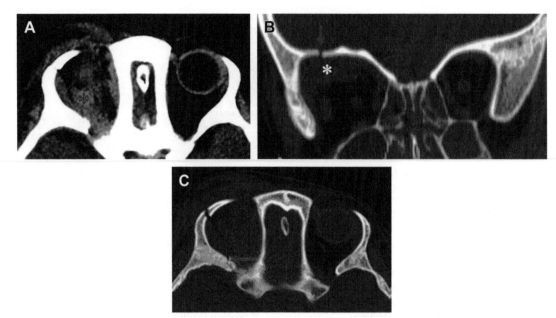

Fig. 9. Orbital hematocyst. Child status post fall. (*A*) Axial CT soft tissue window image and (*B*) coronal bone window CT image show an extraconal hematoma (*asterisk*) underlying an orbital roof fracture (*arrow*). (*C*) Note how the fracture line extends into the right lesser wing of the sphenoid (*arrow*). Because the lateral orbital roof is relatively rigid, fractures tend to propagate into the neurocranium.

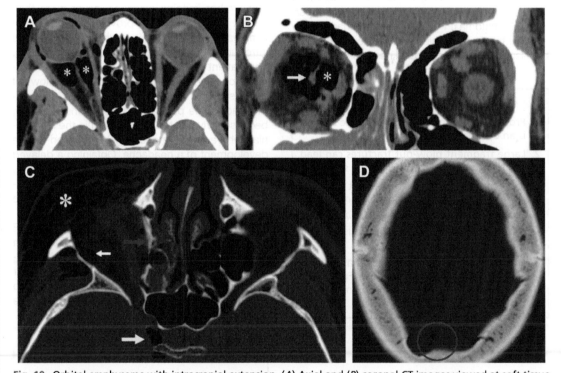

Fig. 10. Orbital emphysema with intracranial extension. (*A*) Axial and (*B*) coronal CT images viewed at soft tissue window demonstrate extensive orbital emphysema (*asterisks*) outlining the optic nerve (*yellow arrow*). Note that this is caused by a small orbital floor fracture (*red arrow*). There is proptosis and abnormal straightening of the optic nerve. The patient underwent a decompression/canthotomy in the emergency room with rapid restoration of vision. (*C, D*) Axial CT images in a different patient demonstrate a medial orbital wall fracture (*red arrow*) and both preseptal (*asterisk*) and postseptal orbital emphysema (*white arrow*). The air extends intravenously into the right cavernous sinus (*yellow arrow*) and into the superficial cortical veins draining to sagittal sinus (*circle*).

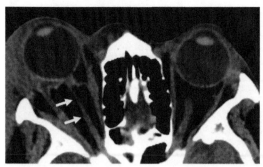

Fig. 11. Globe tethering and increased intraorbital pressure. Axial CT image shows that the posterior aspect of the right globe has lost its normal spherical shape because of proptosis with nerve tethering (*arrows*). In rare cases, the tethering can actually result in separation of the optic nerve from the globe. This elderly female underwent emergent orbital decompression/canthotomy in the emergency room for vision preservation.

MIDFACE FRACTURES

The face is supported by stronger/thickened areas of the facial skeleton termed buttresses. These buttresses confer the facial structures a rigid protective frame. The vertically oriented buttresses are considered stronger than the buttresses oriented horizontally (see **Figs. 1** and **2**).

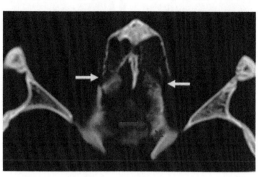

Fig. 12. Comminuted fracture of ethmoids and floor of anterior cranial fossa. Axial CT image shows multiple medial orbital wall fractures (*yellow arrows*). The fracture line (*red arrow*) extends to the left optic canal (*asterisk*) raising concern for optic nerve injury.

Zygomaticomaxillary Complex Fractures

Zygomaticomaxillary complex fractures (ZMC) are second only to fractures of the nasal bone in overall frequency.[1] Previously misnamed the "tripod" fracture, the ZMC fracture is the result of a direct blow to the malar eminence and involves disruption at four sites: (1) the lateral orbital rim, (2) the inferior orbital rim, (3) the zygomaticomaxillary buttress, and (4) the zygomatic arch. The ZMC fracture disrupts all four zygomatic sutures (**Fig. 16**). Fixation plates may be placed across the orbital rim, the sutures, and buttresses (**Fig. 17**). The ZMC fracture may be associated

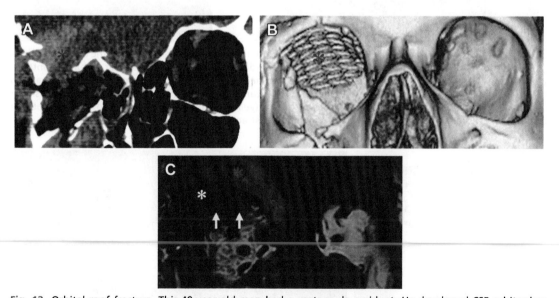

Fig. 13. Orbital roof fracture. This 49-year-old man had a motorcycle accident. He developed CSF orbitorrhea 1 week later. (*A*) Coronal reformation CT viewed at soft tissue window shows intraorbital herniation of a hemorrhagic contusion of right frontal lobe (*asterisk*). (*B*) Three-dimensional reformation illustrates orbital roof reconstruction with a Medpor plate (*asterisk*). (*C*) Coronal magnetic resonance imaging FLAIR sequence demonstrates the vascularized pericranial flap (*yellow asterisk*) placed cephalad to the Medpor plate (*arrows*) to prevent recurrence of CSF leak. The right inferior frontal lobe contusion is identified (*red asterisk*).

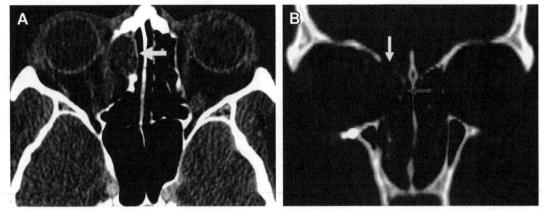

Fig. 14. Posttraumatic meningocele. This 58-year-old man has a history of sinonasal polyposis and a clinical concern for an inverted papilloma. (*A*) Axial CT image viewed at soft tissue window demonstrates an extraconal water attenuation lesion (*arrow*). (*B*) Coronal reformation bone window CT image shows right orbital roof dehiscence (*yellow arrow*) and a remote medial orbital blow-out fracture (*red arrow*). The orbital lesion is consistent with posttraumatic meningocele.

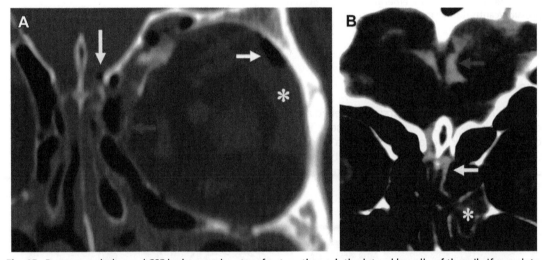

Fig. 15. Pneumocephalus and CSF leak secondary to a fracture through the lateral lamella of the cribriform plate. (*A*) Coned-down coronal nonenhanced view of the left orbit demonstrates a tiny focus of air within the anterior cranial fossa (*yellow arrow*). Also evident is an extraconal hematoma (*asterisk*) and emphysema (*white arrow*) within the lateral left orbit and a medial wall blow-out fracture (*red arrow*). (*B*) Coronal CT cisternogram shows contrast extravasation into the left nasal olfactory recess (*yellow arrow*) and pooling into the left anterior ethmoid air cells (*asterisk*). Intracranial subarachnoid contrast accumulation is also noted (*red arrow*).

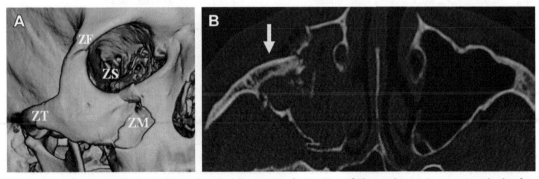

Fig. 16. ZMC fracture. (*A*) Three-dimensional oblique CT reformation of the malar eminence reveals the four zygomatic sutures: zygomaticofrontal (ZF), zygomaticomaxillary (ZM), zygomaticotemporal (ZT), and zygomaticosphenoid (ZS). (*B*) Axial CT image demonstrates the markedly flattened right malar eminence (*arrow*). Acutely, the cosmetic deformity is often clinically unappreciated because of the overlying soft tissue swelling.

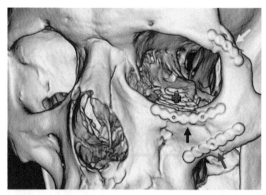

Fig. 17. Postoperative CT in a complex ZMC fracture. Three-dimensional oblique reformatted CT in a patient who underwent open reduction internal fixation (ORIF) for a left ZMC fracture. Note the zygomaticomaxillary (*red arrow*), zygomaticofrontal (*yellow arrow*), and inferior orbital rim (*black arrow*) fractures that have been surgically repaired with monocortical plates and nonlocking screws. The orbital floor fracture was repaired with a reconstruction plate (*red cross*) by a vestibular and transconjunctival approach.

with either increased or decreased volume of the orbit, depending on the direction and rotation of fracture fragments.

Although mildly displaced ZMC fractures can be managed conservatively (if the patient is asymptomatic), displaced fractures should be corrected surgically[11] for prevention of visual impairment and trismus. Trismus typically occurs when a depressed zygomatic arch (**Fig. 18**) compresses the masticator muscles.

Midface fractures often involve the nasolacrimal duct and may result in epiphora. Most commonly, a bypass tube is placed within the native nasolacrimal duct to restore patency.[12] Occasionally, the nasolacrimal duct cannot be salvaged (**Fig. 19**).

Le Fort Fractures

Le Fort fractures are defined by craniofacial dissociation (disjunction), because all Le Fort fractures (I–III) involve the posterior maxillary buttress (see **Fig. 2**) formed by the pterygoid plates, which connect the sphenoid bone (skull base) to the midface.

Many midface fractures do not follow the true Le Fort pattern and are more complex with coexistence of different additional fractures superimposed on Le Fort fractures. However, describing a midface fracture using the Le Fort classification helps summarize and succinctly communicate the midface injury.

Le Fort Fracture Classification	Imaging Clue
Le Fort I: "The floating palate" (Fig. 20)	Involvement of nasal aperture
Le Fort II: "The floating maxilla" (Fig. 21)	Fracture through inferior orbital rim
Le Fort III: "The floating face" (Fig. 22)	Involvement of zygomatic arch

Recognition of the Le Fort pattern by a single specific area involved can be helpful: Le Fort I, the anterolateral margin of the nasal fossa; Le Fort II, the inferior orbital rim; and Le Fort III, the zygomatic arch.[13] However, more complex fractures may occur and Le Fort II and III can coexist on the same side of the face.

Given the severity of injury, a screening CT angiogram of the neck is recommended and should be performed in Le Fort II and III fractures to exclude blunt traumatic neck arterial dissections.[14]

Nasal Bones and Septum

Nasal bone fractures are the most common facial fractures encountered in the daily emergency room imaging for trauma[1] because of the protrusion of this relatively thin bone (**Fig. 23**).

Immediately after trauma, before edema ensues, a closed reduction of nasal fractures may be performed. Open reduction is reserved for comminuted fractures with loss of nasal support, severe septal injuries, and marked soft tissue

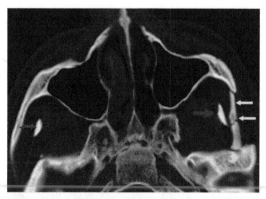

Fig. 18. Comminuted and depressed fracture of left zygomatic arch. Axial CT demonstrates flattening of the left zygomatic arch (*yellow arrows*). The fragments are displaced against the coronoid process (*red arrow*) of the mandible. Compare with the distance between the normal right coronoid process and the zygomatic arch (*double-headed arrow*). Compression of masticator muscles by the zygomatic arch fracture fragments results in trismus.

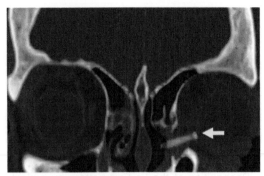

Fig. 19. Dacryocystorhinostomy. Coronal CT examination demonstrates bypass of the normal lacrimal drainage pathway by a Jones tube (*arrow*) surgically placed to drain into the middle nasal meatus in a case of traumatic nasolacrimal duct injury.

damage. Delayed surgical intervention after the initial swelling subsides is considered adequate if circumstances prevent acute correction. The deformity correction is necessary for restoration of function of the nasal passages,[15] because a turbulent nasal cavity air flow may lead to sinusitis. Sinusitis may also occur if a bone fragment is displaced into the maxillary sinus.

Nasal septal hematomas must be addressed acutely to prevent cartilaginous pressure necrosis and a subsequent "saddle-nose" deformity. In addition, untreated hematomas can result in abscess formation. A large nasal septal hematoma may be evident on CT (**Fig. 24**), but the diagnosis is usually made clinically.

Naso-Orbito-Ethmoid Fractures

Imaging of nasal bone fractures is considered optional, unless significant trauma has occurred

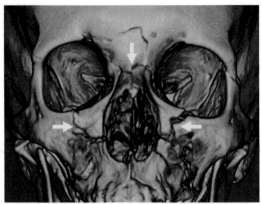

Fig. 21. The Le Fort II fracture. Coronal three-dimensional reformatted CT image demonstrates a triangular-shaped fracture (*arrows*) traversing across the maxilla leaving a larger portion of the maxilla and nasal aperture in the inferior fragment. The fracture characteristically involves the inferior orbital rims, separates the nose and inferior maxilla from the lateral midface, and involves the nasofrontal suture. Note that the medial maxillary sinus wall is spared in the Le Fort II fracture.

with involvement of the proximal nasal bones. These fractures can extend to the frontal bone and the cribriform plate, involve the midface and orbit, and are named naso-orbito-ethmoid (NOE) fractures. The NOE fractures are complex because they can be associated with intracranial and orbital injuries and a head and face CT scan is warranted. NOE fracture frequency has markedly decreased since the universal use of airbags, and reportedly currently account for approximately 5% of adult and 15% of pediatric facial fractures.[16]

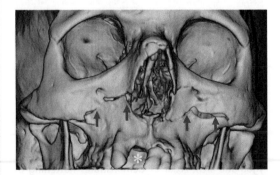

Fig. 20. The Le Fort I fracture. Coronal three-dimensional reformatted CT image demonstrates a transverse maxillary fracture traversing through the maxillary antrum and the nasal cavity above the nasal floor (*arrows*). This horizontal fracture characteristically extends into the lateral wall of the nasal aperture. Avulsion of the right incisors is also noted (*asterisk*).

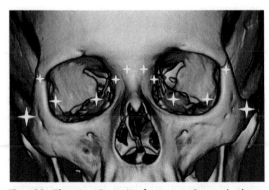

Fig. 22. The Le Fort III fracture. Coronal three-dimensional CT shows a horizontal fracture traversing the lateral and medial orbits (*small stars*) to separate the cranium from the face. The zygomatic arches (*large stars*) are characteristically involved.

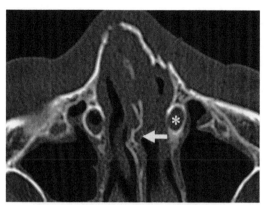

Fig. 23. Comminuted nasal-septal fracture. Axial CT demonstrates rightward nasal deviation and a comminuted left nasal bone fracture (*red arrow*) and buckled osseous nasal septum (*yellow arrow*). The nasolacrimal duct is intact (*asterisk*).

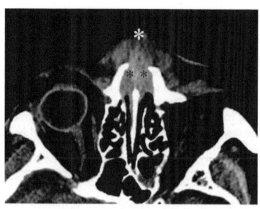

Fig. 24. Upper nasal septal hematoma in a patient with nasal bone fractures. Noncontrast axial CT demonstrates extensive anterior nasal soft tissue swelling (*yellow asterisk*) and hyperdense soft tissue (*red asterisks*) on both sides of nasal septum. The septal hematoma in this elderly man was managed conservatively.

NOE injuries are divided in three groups according to the degree of injury to the medial canthal attachment using the Manson classification:

Manson classification of NOE fractures
Type I: Single fragment (most common) (Fig. 25A).
Type II: Comminuted with intact insertion of medial canthal tendon.
Type III: Comminuted with lateral displacement or avulsion of medial canthal ligament (uncommon).

The most important factor in determining the need for surgical correction of NOE injury is stability of the bone to which the medial canthal tendon attaches. The medial canthal tendon inserts at the most anterior aspect of medial orbital wall. Although comminution of medial orbital rim and wall can be assessed radiographically, avulsion of the medial canthal tendon is best diagnosed clinically under anesthesia. A mobile fracture at the insertion of medial canthal tendon or avulsion of the tendon results in telecanthus.

Additionally, NOE fracture is commonly associated with nasolacrimal canal fracture (see Fig. 25B). The CT report should mention this injury

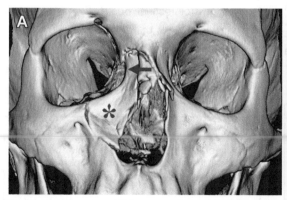

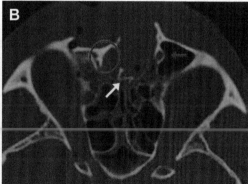

Fig. 25. NOE fracture. (*A*) Large medial orbit rim fragment (*asterisk*) usually implies preserved insertion of right medial canthal tendon. Note involvement with depression at the right nasofrontal suture (*red arrow*). (*B*) The area of the right nasolacrimal duct (*circled*) is severely distorted (compare with the normal left nasolacrimal canal [*red arrow*]). The osseous nasal septum is buckled posteriorly (*yellow arrow*). This substance abuse patient deferred treatment and, to date, has not undergone surgical repair.

because it may not be clinically apparent early on and patients may develop epiphora and/or recurrent dacryocystorhinitis.

Inadequate treatment may result in difficult-to-treat secondary deformities. Severely comminuted fractures require repositioning of the medial canthal tendon.[17] The nasal septum plays an important role as a central sagittal buttress and must be restored for successful surgical repair of NOE fracture and nasal depression.[18]

Key points: midface fractures

1. Most frequent midface fractures involve the nasal bone, followed by fractures affecting the ZMC.

2. With Le Fort II and III injury, strong consideration should be given to CT angiogram of the neck to exclude vascular injury.

3. The radiology report should include the status of the medial orbital rim, because its comminution implies involvement of the medial canthal tendon.

4. Fracture fragments within the maxillary sinus should be noted because they may function as a nidus for infection.

5. Nasolacrimal duct involvement may lead to epiphora, dacryocystocele, and dacryocystitis.

DENTAL

Tooth injuries are frequently identified on CT scans of the face. At times it may be difficult to clearly distinguish periodontal disease from dental injury, but evaluation of adjacent teeth would provide a clue to the overall dental health.

Andreasen and colleagues[19] described dental trauma as divided into nine fracture and six luxation entities, but with as many as 54 combination injuries in which both luxation and fracture occur. These complex injuries have distinct healing scenarios for which treatment consensus is still a work in progress. The main traumatic entities identified on imaging are as follows:

Dental trauma classification

1. Intrusion

2. Extrusion (Fig. 26)

3. Lateral luxation

4. Crown fracture

5. Root fracture

6. Crown/root fracture (Fig. 27)

7. Avulsion (see Fig. 26; Fig. 28)

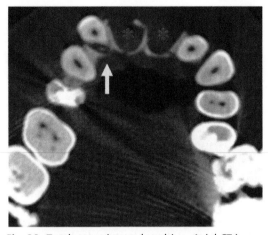

Fig. 26. Tooth extrusion and avulsion. Axial CT image shows the right lateral maxillary incisor is extruded (*arrow* points to periapical lucency) and the central incisors are avulsed (*asterisks*).

Alveolar ridge fractures (see **Fig. 28**) are considered open fractures and require, besides splinting, an antibiotic regimen.

Once a tooth avulsion is identified, scrutiny of neck and chest films for the aspirated tooth should be performed. An avulsed tooth in the airway/upper aerodigestive tract (**Fig. 29**) must be retrieved because aspirated foreign bodies within the small airways can lead to obstructive pneumonia, and even abscess formation. Tooth aspiration is reportedly more common in children. If the patient is intubated, a flexible bronchoscope is introduced through the orotracheal tube for safe foreign body retrieval.

Once in the esophagus, the avulsed tooth need not be retrieved because a high proportion of accidentally ingested teeth are passed in the stool within 1 month. Only a minority of ingested teeth lead to gastrointestinal obstruction, perforation, or bleeding.

Initiation of treatment of injured teeth, either primary or permanent, has the best outcome if performed within 1 hour to prevent pulp necrosis and loss of bone.

Key points: dental trauma

1. Alveolar ridge fractures should be noted because they are treated as open fractures and patients are placed on an antibiotic regimen.

2. Scrutiny of chest and neck images for aspiration of an avulsed tooth should be performed because aspirated teeth may cause pneumonia and lung abscess.

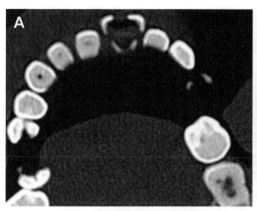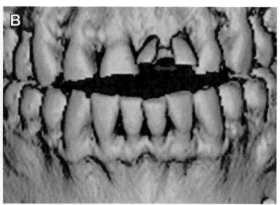

Fig. 27. Crown fracture. (A) Axial and (B) three-dimensional coronal reformatted CT images show a fracture of the left maxillary central incisor crown and root (not shown) with splaying of fracture fragments (arrow). The patient underwent dental extraction.

MANDIBLE

As described previously with the midface, the mandible also has its own buttresses (ie, areas of strong, thickened facial bone areas) (Fig. 30). These are similarly important for surgical repair planning.

Mandibular fractures are most commonly bilateral. A symphyseal or body fracture is typically associated with a contralateral angle or subcondylar neck fracture (Fig. 31). The angle fracture frequently traverses the root of the third molar.

The surgical approach is first directed toward repair of the anterior (teeth-bearing, symphysis,

and body) mandible before reducing the posterior segment (angle, ramus, coronoid, and condyle). "Intermaxillary" (maxillomandibular) fixation is often the first step in repair of mandibular fractures (Fig. 32C, D).

Subcondylar Fractures and Condylar Dislocations

Closed treatment of subcondylar fractures through maxillomandibular fixation, even when associated with condylar dislocation (Fig. 33), has been advocated as prudent given the occurrence of complications with open surgery (salivary fistula, facial nerve paresis, and so

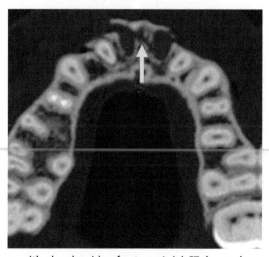

Fig. 28. Avulsed central incisors with alveolar ridge fracture. Axial CT shows absence of the maxillary central incisors and a fracture through the alveolar ridge (arrow).

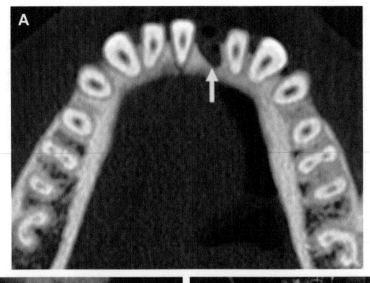

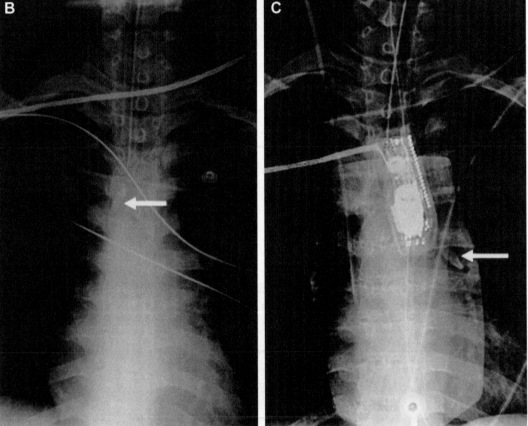

Fig. 29. Avulsed left central incisor. (*A*) Axial CT demonstrates absence of the left central incisor (*arrow*). Note the lucency around the apex of right central incisor suggesting an extrusion. (*B*) Anteroposterior chest radiographs reveal the missing tooth identified first in the trachea (*arrow*), and then (*C*) the left mainstem bronchus (*arrow*). The patient underwent bronchoscopy with successful tooth retrieval.

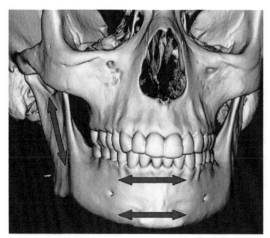

Fig. 30. Mandibular buttresses: upper, lower, and vertical (*arrows*).

As in Le Fort II and II fractures, screening CT angiography of the neck is recommended in the setting of condylar fractures with dislocaton. The CT angiogram is recommended to exclude internal carotid dissection or pseudoaneurysm.[14]

Coronoid Process Fractures

Conservative management is also used for fractures of the coronoid process when there is minimal displacement and no restriction of mouth opening. For patients with significant fracture displacement and limited mouth opening, or patients with concomitant fractures of the zygoma, zygomatic arch, or mandibular ramus, ORIF is often used.[24]

forth).[20] Either open or closed reduction is chosen based on severity of comminution of condylar head and, most importantly, function impairment.[21,22] Open reduction internal fixation (ORIF) is becoming increasingly favored because endoscope-assisted ORIF is gaining ground.[23] The closed treatment approach for condylar fractures and dislocations is commonly chosen in children, unless function is severely impaired.

Quite frequently, the condyle is driven posteriorly into the external auditory canal by a blow or a fall onto the chin (**Fig. 34**).

Key points: mandible trauma

1. The anterior (teeth-bearing) mandibular fractures are corrected first, typically by ORIF.

2. The alignment of the posterior segment (angle, ramus, and condyle) is subsequently corrected, most commonly by closed intermaxillary (maxillomandibular) fixation.

3. Condylar fracture dislocations are an indication for CT angiogram of neck to evaluate for vascular injury (dissection).

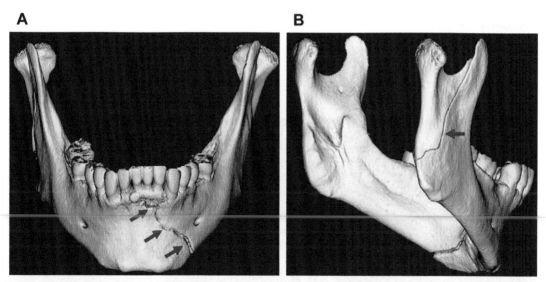

Fig. 31. Parasymphyseal fracture with extension into the alveolar ridge with en block mobility of mandibular incisors and contralateral posterior segment (subcondylar) fracture. (*A*) Isolated three-dimensional coronal CT reformatted image of the mandible demonstrates an oblique fracture line extending to the alveolar ridge fracture (*arrows*). (*B*) Three-dimensional posterior oblique reformatted CT image demonstrates the contralateral ramus fracture extending to the mandibular angle (*arrow*).

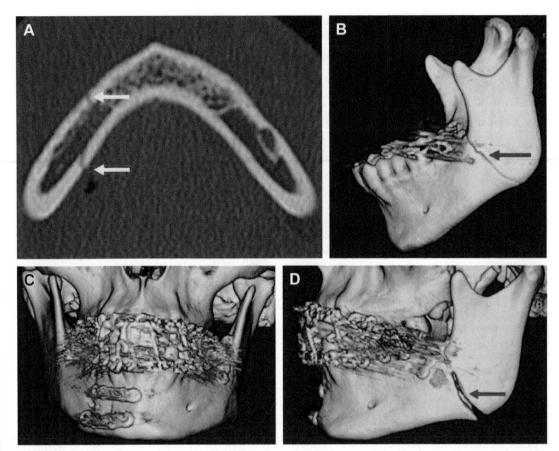

Fig. 32. Bilateral mandibular fractures and surgical repair. (*A, B*) Common bilateral fracture pattern of mandibular fractures. In this case linear fractures are seen in the right parasymphyseal region (*yellow arrows*) and the left mandibular angle (*red arrow*). (*C, D*) Mandibulomaxillary wire and arch bar fixation with right parasymphyseal plate and screw placement. Note the extensive postoperative beam-hardening artifact obscuring optimal visualization of the alveolar region. There is mild diastasis of the left mandibular angle fracture (*arrow*), which was subsequently corrected.

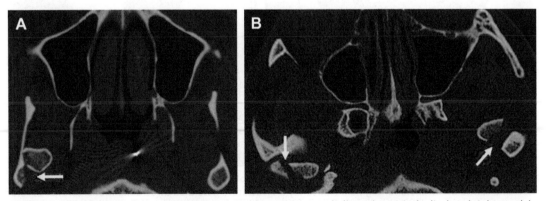

Fig. 33. Condylar fracture dislocation. (*A*). Axial CT demonstrates medially and anteriorly displaced right condylar fracture (*arrow*). (*B*) Axial CT in a different patient reveals bilateral distracted condylar fractures and left condylar dislocation (*arrows*). This patient underwent closed intermaxillary fixation.

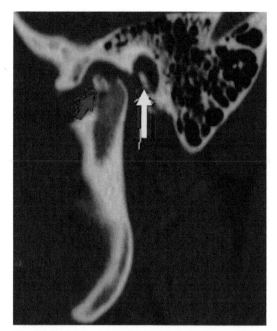

Fig. 34. Fractured condyle with anterior wall of external auditory canal fracture and posterior displacement. Parasagittal CT through the temporomandibular joint shows a fracture of the anterior wall of the external auditory canal (*yellow arrow*) caused by traumatic impact from the mandibular condyle. Note the mandibular condyle is also fractured (*red arrow*).

SUMMARY

Knowledge of typical patterns of facial fractures is important because each pattern may be associated with its respective functional complications. The three-dimensional images are commonly used by surgeons for operative planning in restoration of alignment and correction of cosmetic deformities, but can be occasionally useful to the radiologist as a summary view of complex midface fractures.

REFERENCES

1. Allareddy V, Allareddy V, Nalliah RP. Epidemiology of facial fracture injuries. J Oral Maxillofac Surg 2011; 69(10):2613–8.
2. Bell RB, Dierks EJ, Brar P, et al. A protocol for the management of frontal sinus fractures emphasizing sinus preservation. J Oral Maxillofac Surg 2007; 65(5):825–39.
3. Metzinger SE, Guerra AB, Garcia RE. Frontal sinus fractures: management guidelines. Facial Plast Surg 2005;21(3):199–206.
4. Donath A, Sindwani R. Frontal sinus cranialization using the pericranial flap: an added layer of protection. Laryngoscope 2006;116(9):1585–8.
5. Cole P, Kaufman Y, Momoh A, et al. Techniques in frontal sinus fracture repair. Plast Reconstr Surg 2009;123(5):1578–9.
6. Echo A, Troy JS, Hollier LH Jr. Frontal sinus fractures. Semin Plast Surg 2010;24(4):375–82.
7. Shah HA, Shipchandler TZ, Sufyan AS, et al. Use of fracture size and soft tissue herniation on computed tomography to predict diplopia in isolated orbital floor fractures. Am J Otolaryngol 2013;34:695–8.
8. Wang DH, Zheng CQ, Qian J, et al. Endoscopic optic nerve decompression for the treatment of traumatic optic nerve neuropathy. ORL J Otorhinolaryngol Relat Spec 2008;70(2):130–3.
9. Levin LA, Beck RW, Joseph MP, et al. The treatment of traumatic optic neuropathy: the International Optic Nerve Trauma Study. Ophthalmology 1999; 106(7):1268–77.
10. Bell RB, Dierks EJ, Homer L, et al. Management of cerebrospinal fluid leak associated with craniomaxillofacial trauma. J Oral Maxillofac Surg 2004;62(6): 676–84.
11. Pau CY, Barrera JE, Kwon J, et al. Three-dimensional analysis of zygomatic-maxillary complex fracture patterns. Craniomaxillofac Trauma Reconstr 2010;3(3):167–76.
12. Watkins LM, Janfaza P, Rubin PA. The evolution of endonasal dacryocystorhinostomy. Surv Ophthalmol 2003;48(1):73–84.
13. Rhea JT, Novelline RA. How to simplify the CT diagnosis of Le Fort fractures. Am J Roentgenol 2005; 184(5):1700–5.
14. Schneidereit NP, Simons R, Nicolaou S, et al. Utility of screening for blunt vascular neck injuries with computed tomographic angiography. J Trauma 2006;60(1):209–15.
15. Kelley BP, Downey CR, Stal S. Evaluation and reduction of nasal trauma. Semin Plast Surg 2010;24(4): 339–47.
16. Nguyen M, Koshy JC, Hollier LH Jr. Pearls of nasoorbitoethmoid trauma management. Semin Plast Surg 2010;24(4):383–8.
17. Herford AS, Ying T, Brown B. Outcomes of severely comminuted (type III) nasoorbitoethmoid fractures. J Oral Maxillofac Surg 2005;63(9):1266–77.
18. Yabe T, Ozawa T. Treatment of nasoethmoid-orbital fractures using Kirschner wire fixation of the nasal septum. J Craniofac Surg 2011;22(4): 1510–2.
19. Andreasen JO, Lauridsen E, Gerds TA, et al. Dental trauma guide: a source of evidence-based treatment guidelines for dental trauma. Dent Traumatol 2012;28(2):142–7.
20. Pal US, Singh RK, Dhasmana S, et al. Use of 3-D plate in displaced angle fracture of mandible. Craniomaxillofac Trauma Reconstr 2013;6(1): 25–30.

21. Chrcanovic BR. Open versus closed reduction: diacapitular fractures of the mandibular condyle. Oral Maxillofac Surg 2012;16(3):257–65.

22. Eckelt U, Schneider M, Erasmus F, et al. Open versus closed treatment of fractures of the mandibular condylar process-a prospective randomized multi-centre study. J Craniomaxillofac Surg 2006;34(5):306–14.

23. Abdel-Galil K, Loukota R. Fractures of the mandibular condyle: evidence base and current concepts of management. Br J Oral Maxillofac Surg 2010; 48(7):520–6.

24. Shen L, Li J, Li P, et al. Mandibular coronoid fractures: treatment options. Int J Oral Maxillofac Surg 2013;42(6):721–6.

Orbital Soft-Tissue Trauma

J. Levi Chazen, MD[a],*, Joshua Lantos, MD[a], Ajay Gupta, MD[a], Gary J. Lelli Jr, MD[b], C. Douglas Phillips, MD[a],*

KEYWORDS

- Orbits • Trauma • Computed tomography • Magnetic resonance imaging • Imaging • Soft tissue

KEY POINTS

- Significant morbidity is associated with orbital trauma, including permanent visual loss.
- In the clinical assessment of orbital trauma, visual acuity and extraocular muscle motility are critical for rapid evaluation of injury severity.
- Assessment of these parameters may be limited by edema and concomitant injuries.
- Imaging may further delineate the trauma pattern and extent of injury, and is performed early and often in patients with significant orbital trauma.

IMAGING TECHNIQUES

In patients with orbital trauma, physical examination and history should focus on rapid evaluation of injury severity. Mechanism and timing of injury may provide valuable clinical information in the workup of such patients. Visual acuity testing, intraocular pressure, slit-lamp examination with fluorescein and fundoscopy are helpful for assessment, but may be limited if severe trauma is present or globe rupture is suspected. Visual acuity and extraocular motility are the 2 most important functions to be evaluated emergently.[1] Evaluation of these clinical parameters may be limited by edema and concomitant injuries. Imaging may further delineate the trauma pattern and extent of injury, and is performed early and often in patients with significant orbital trauma.

ORBITAL ANATOMY

Familiarity with normal orbital anatomy is important for the interpretation of trauma studies (**Fig. 1**). The globe is a spherical 2- to 3-cm structure with 3 concentric layers: the outer sclera, the vascular choroid, and inner retina, continuous with the optic nerve. The sclera blends into the cornea and is covered by the translucent conjunctiva ventrally. The uvea describes the middle layer and consists of the choroid, ciliary body, and iris. The globe can be separated into the anterior and posterior segments by the lens. The anterior segment is further subdivided into the anterior and posterior chamber by the iris; aqueous humor is produced by the ciliary body and flows to the anterior chamber. The lens is suspended by zonule fibers, and muscular contractions of the ciliary body result in lens deformity. The posterior segment contains gelatinous vitreous humor.

CHOICE OF IMAGING

Radiology plays a critical role in the diagnosis and treatment planning of traumatic orbital injuries. Imaging may be indicated if the posterior chamber is not visualized on ophthalmologic examination, or if there is clinical concern for orbital fracture, intraocular foreign body, or occult globe rupture.[2]

Disclosures: None.
[a] Department of Radiology, Weill Cornell Medical College, 525 East 68th Street, New York, NY 10065, USA;
[b] Department of Ophthalmology, Weill Cornell Medical College, 525 East 68th Street, New York, NY 10065, USA
* Corresponding authors. Department of Radiology, Weill Cornell Medical College, 525 East 68th Street, Starr 8A, Box 141, New York, NY 10065.
E-mail addresses: jlc2008@med.cornell.edu; cdp2001@med.cornell.edu

Neuroimag Clin N Am 24 (2014) 425–437
http://dx.doi.org/10.1016/j.nic.2014.03.005
1052-5149/14/$ – see front matter © 2014 Elsevier Inc. All rights reserved.

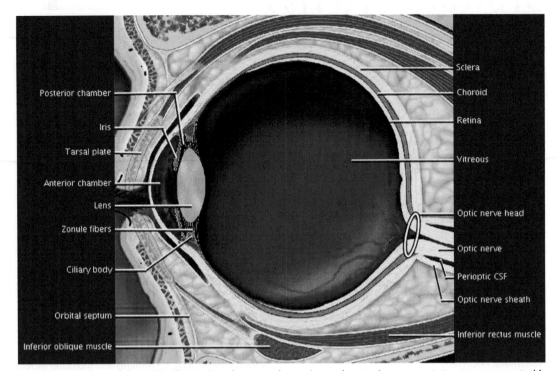

Fig. 1. Sagittal view of the orbit, illustrating the normal anterior and posterior segment structures separated by the lens. The 3 layers of the orbit are illustrated: outer sclera, vascular choroid, and inner retina. CSF, cerebrospinal fluid. (*Courtesy of* Amirsys Inc, Salt Lake City (UT); with permission.)

Computed tomography (CT) is typically the first-line modality, given its rapid acquisition and availability; however, other modalities may have distinct advantages.

Radiography

The role of conventional radiographs has diminished significantly, given the current availability of CT. Standard Caldwell (orbitofrontal view; beam tilted 15–20° caudal) and Waters (occipitomental view; chin raised) views have sensitivities ranging from 64% to 78% for detection of orbital fractures, with false-negative findings in 9% to 29%.[3] Given the moderate sensitivity and false negatives, plain films have limited clinical utility.

Computed Tomography

CT has become the first-line imaging study in patients with ocular trauma.[4] Rapid acquisition and thin-section multiplanar reformations of CT allow for accurate assessment of orbital fracture and associated injuries.[1] CT demonstrates a high sensitivity for fracture detection that is optimized by thin-section acquisition, multiplanar reformations, and 3-dimensional modeling.[5] Furthermore, for polytrauma cranial evaluation can be performed concurrently with CT imaging.

Although CT is very sensitive for detection of orbital fracture, its accuracy in soft-tissue injuries may be more limited. In a study from 2000, CT demonstrated 73% sensitivity and 95% specificity for the detection of open-globe injury.[6] Magnetic resonance (MR) imaging holds significant advantages for the assessment of retinal and choroidal detachments and nonradiopaque foreign bodies.

The lens is a radiosensitive organ, and efforts should be made to limit the radiation delivered. Modern multidetector helical CT scanning techniques demonstrate significant benefit in dose reduction over older single-detector setups. There is evidence that limiting the tube current to 100 mA instead of the conventional 300 mA setting may decrease the effective dose by 70% without compromising detection of traumatic injury.[7]

Ultrasonography

Ultrasonography can be performed rapidly at the bedside, and appears to provide accurate detection of retrobulbar hemorrhage, foreign body, lens dislocation, and retinal detachment.[8] However, it is contraindicated in the setting of globe rupture because of the pressure applied during sonographic assessment, possibly exacerbating an unstable globe.[8,9] Although ultrasonography is limited in the assessment of complex facial fractures, it appears to provide accuracy comparable with that of CT in the detection of fractures of the infraorbital rim and orbital floor.[10]

MR Imaging

In the acute presentation of ocular trauma, MR imaging has limited utility because of its longer acquisition time and decreased sensitivity for fracture in comparison with CT. Furthermore, MR imaging is contraindicated if a metallic ocular foreign body is suspected.[9] MR imaging holds significant advantages in the detection of organic foreign bodies (eg, wood).[2]

ANTERIOR CHAMBER INJURIES

The anterior chamber is located between the cornea and iris and contains aqueous fluid. Clinically and by imaging, the anterior chamber should be assessed for the presence of abnormal material (eg, blood, foreign body) and abnormal depth. Deepening of the anterior chamber may result from lens dislocation, scleral rupture, or iridodialysis (rupture of the iris–ciliary body attachments). The anterior chamber may be abnormally shallow as a result of lens dislocation, corneal injury, choroidal hemorrhage, or acute angle closure.[2]

Anterior chamber depth (ACD) on CT appears to correspond with open-globe injury. An asymmetric difference in ACD of 0.4 mm or greater has 73% sensitivity and 100% specificity for detection of open-globe injury.[11] Corneal laceration may result in decreased ACD (**Fig. 2**) and may be accompanied by iris prolapse. Anterior lens dislocation may mimic traumatic corneal laceration, and the lens should be carefully examined.[12]

Traumatic Hyphema

A traumatic hyphema is caused by bleeding in the anterior chamber secondary to disruption of blood vessels in the iris or ciliary body.[9] A blood-aqueous level may be apparent on inspection, and increased intraocular pressure may result. Rebleeding may occur in 20% of patients, typically 2 to 5 days following injury when the initial clot retracts. Clinically it is important to assess for a bleeding diathesis, such as sickle cell disease, which can significantly increase the severity of the hyphema and the likelihood and rate of rebleed.[8] Hyphema may be classified in 4 grades, the most significant being an "8-ball hyphema" resulting from an anterior chamber completely filled with hemorrhage. More than half of traumatic hyphemas are the result of sports-related injuries.[13] Imaging is not required for the diagnosis of traumatic hyphema

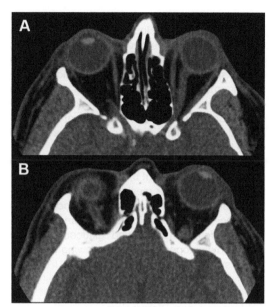

Fig. 2. (A, B) Axial noncontrast computed tomography (CT). Corneal laceration resulting in decreased anterior chamber depth in the left eye (B). Note that the normal density of the lens is preserved.

but is frequently performed to assess for more significant injury. The hyphema is manifested on orbital CT by increased attenuation in the anterior chamber. Disruption of these same iris and ciliary vessels may result in bleeding into the posterior chamber, a vitreous hemorrhage (see later discussion).

Subconjunctival Hemorrhage

Subconjunctival hemorrhage may occur from minor trauma such as sneezing, coughing, or Valsalva, and results from tearing of small subconjunctival blood vessels. The dramatic appearance may bring patients to medical attention when a painless, red conjunctival lesion is evident. The area should not be raised, and visual acuity should be preserved. Cross-sectional imaging is not necessary, and the hemorrhage is self-limited.[8]

INJURY TO IRIS AND CILIARY BODIES

Injuries to the iris and ciliary bodies are typically assessed on clinical examination. Thorough evaluation of the iris and ciliary body is performed with a mirror/prism (gonioscope) in conjunction with a slit lamp to evaluate the iridocorneal angle.[14] Cross-sectional imaging may be normal, unless associated vascular injury is present with anterior and/or posterior chamber hemorrhage.

Traumatic iridocyclitis results from blunt trauma to the iris and ciliary body that may cause spasm and blurry vision. This condition is typically self-limited; short-term cycloplegic (dilating and paralyzing) therapy may be given. Traumatic mydriasis and miosis result from similar traumatic injury to the iris sphincter. Although this condition is self-limited, imaging may be performed to exclude cranial nerve injury as the underlying cause.[8] Traumatic iridodialysis is the result of a tear in the peripheral iris resulting in separation of the iris and ciliary body.

Glaucoma can result from traumatic obstruction of aqueous outflow from blood (hyphema), disruption of the trabecular meshwork, or lens dislocation. Delayed-onset glaucoma can occur from angle recession, lens dislocation, or various hemolytic manifestations. Delayed glaucoma is also seen following open-globe injury, owing to formation of synechiae.[14]

LENS INJURIES
Subluxation and Dislocation

The zonule fibers responsible for holding the lens in place may be disrupted by blunt trauma, resulting in lens detachment. Patients will clinically display blurred vision, monocular diplopia, or distortion if partial lens dislocation is present. Most commonly the lens will dislocate posteriorly because the iris prevents anterior translation. However, anterior lens dislocations can occur, and may mimic decreased ACD caused by corneal laceration. Anterior lens dislocation may also result in acute angle closure glaucoma by mechanical obstruction of aqueous outflow, a condition requiring emergent ophthalmologic attention.[15]

With complete dislocation, the lens is typically displaced posteriorly and lies dependently within the vitreous humor (Fig. 3). When the zonule fibers partially tear, there is asymmetric displacement of the lens away from the ruptured ciliary attachments and posterior displacement into the vitreous humor (Fig. 4).[9]

Trauma is the most common cause of lens dislocation, but bilateral nontraumatic subluxations may be seen with Ehlers-Danlos syndrome, Weill-Marchesani syndrome, aniridia, homocystinuria, and Marfan syndrome.[16]

Traumatic Cataract

The lens capsule normally maintains a dehydrated environment. When the capsule is disrupted, the lens may absorb fluid and swell. This condition manifests clinically as a cloudy edematous lens and is demonstrated on CT by unilateral lens hypoattenuation, a finding specific for traumatic cataract (Fig. 5). A decrease in attenuation of 30 HU

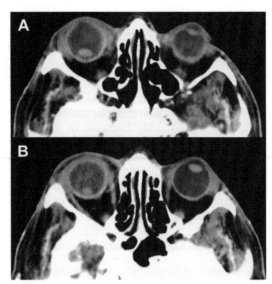

Fig. 3. (A, B) Axial noncontrast CT. Complete dislocation of the right lens following trauma. The dislocated right lens lies dependently within the vitreous humor.

may be seen in the abnormal lens. Treatment is surgical lens replacement.[8] The pathophysiology of traumatic cataract is similar to that of osmotic cataract seen with hyperglycemia, in which elevated glucose in the aqueous humor creates an osmotic gradient that draws fluid into the lens; however, this finding is bilateral in diabetic hyperglycemia.[17]

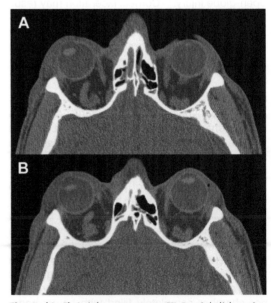

Fig. 4. (A, B) Axial noncontrast CT. Partial dislocation of the right lens is evident, with rupture of the medial zonule fibers and lateral and slight posterior displacement of the lens. The left lens appears normal.

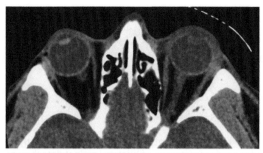

Fig. 5. Axial noncontrast CT. Corneal laceration and decreased left anterior chamber depth with traumatic cataract. When the lens capsule is disrupted, a traumatic cataract results from a swollen edematous lens with low density on CT.

GLOBE INJURIES
Globe Rupture

Open-globe injury, or globe rupture, is a surgical emergency because of the risk of endophthalmitis and the associated high rate of monocular blindness. The standard practice of ophthalmologists worldwide is to undertake a primary surgical repair to restore the structural integrity of the globe. This action is best undertaken at the earliest opportunity, regardless of the extent of the injury and the presenting visual acuity.[18] Although diagnosis of an open-globe injury is obvious when intraocular contents are visualized on ophthalmologic examination, it can be challenging when a patient is unable or unwilling to cooperate, or if severe facial injuries make examination unsafe.[6]

CT is the imaging test of choice for the diagnosis of an open-globe injury and assessment for associated injuries. Findings include a change in globe contour with an obvious loss of volume ("flat-tire" sign), scleral discontinuity, intraocular air, and intraocular foreign body (Figs. 6 and 7).[9] Absent or dislocated lens, vitreous hemorrhage, and retinal detachment are additional predictors of open-globe injury.[19] In a review of 46 patients who underwent surgical exploration, moderate to

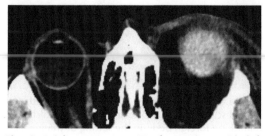

Fig. 6. Axial noncontrast CT of a patient with left facial trauma and left globe volume loss. Total vitreous hemorrhage is present and the lens is absent, both specific for open-globe injury.

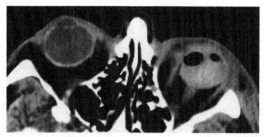

Fig. 7. Axial noncontrast CT of a patient with left facial trauma shows an obvious loss of volume of the left globe, contour change, intraocular gas, and hemorrhage.

severe change in globe contour (flattening or concavity of the sclera in at least 1 quadrant), obvious volume loss, total vitreous hemorrhage, and absence of lens were seen only in eyes with globe rupture.[19]

CT has historically been an imperfect diagnostic modality for ruptured globe. A retrospective review of 200 patients from 1989 to 1993 found that CT had sensitivity of 75% and specificity of 93% for the diagnosis of open-globe injury in the absence of clinical information.[6] In the setting of massive subconjunctival and/or anterior chamber hemorrhage precluding adequate clinical examination in 59 patients, sensitivity was found to be 70%.[20] Sensitivity may be especially limited in the setting of equivocal clinical examination. A review of 46 patients found that when analysis was limited to patients with clinically occult globe rupture, sensitivity decreased from 71% to a range of 56% to 68% between observers, with a negative predictive value of 42% to 50%.[19]

Recent literature, however, suggests better performance for CT when certain findings are considered. Kim and colleagues[11] found 92% sensitivity, 85% specificity, and 89% accuracy for globe rupture in 56 patients when 1 or more of the following are present: change in ACD; change in globe contour; obvious loss of globe volume; dislocated/deformed lens; intraocular foreign body/air; or intraocular hemorrhage. The key finding among these factors was change in ACD. An earlier study reported increased ACD in globe rupture, thought to result from posterior scleral injury decompressing the vitreous, allowing for retropulsion of the lens and deepening of the anterior chamber.[21] However, Kim and colleagues[11] found that 13 of 15 patients (86%) with globe rupture had decreased ACD, a result of either corneal perforation with collapse of the anterior chamber or increased intraocular pressure from hemorrhage (Fig. 8). Regardless of whether ACD increased or decreased, any difference between globes

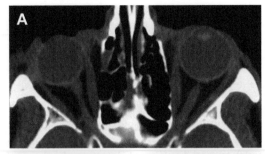

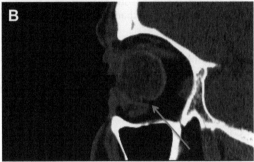

Fig. 8. (A) Axial noncontrast CT of a patient with right facial trauma shows asymmetric decreased right anterior chamber depth, which can result from either corneal perforation or increased intraocular pressure. (B) Medial scleral discontinuity of the right globe (*arrow*) is compatible with globe rupture, also shown at the inferior margin of the right globe on sagittal CT reconstruction.

0.4 mm or larger had 73% sensitivity and 100% specificity for globe rupture.

Potential pitfalls in the diagnosis of open-globe injury include nontraumatic causes of globe-contour deformity, mimics of intraocular air, and mimics of traumatic foreign body. Nontraumatic causes of globe-contour deformity include orbital mass or hematoma, buphthalmos, staphyloma, and coloboma (Fig. 9).[9,16] Mimics of intraocular air include gas injection into the vitreous to tamponade the retina in the treatment of retinal detachment (Fig. 10).[16] Mimics of traumatic foreign

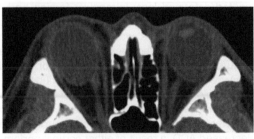

Fig. 9. Axial noncontrast CT of a patient with abnormal contour of the globe secondary to staphylomas. The bilateral nature of this finding helps to exclude open-globe injury. The right lens was normal but out of the imaging plane.

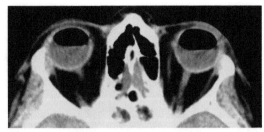

Fig. 10. Axial noncontrast CT of a patient with intraocular gas for treatment of bilateral retinal detachment. The pressure created by injected gas creates a tamponade, forcing the retina into choroid apposition.

body include scleral banding (Fig. 11), silicone oil (Fig. 12), eyelid implants, and glaucoma drainage devices.[22] Surgical history and knowledge of characteristic findings can help suggest the correct diagnosis.

Globe Luxation

Globe luxation, or anterior dislocation of the globe beyond retracted eyelids, results from an extreme proptosis that allows the lids to slip behind the globe equator. It places traction on the optic nerve and retinal vasculature, making early reduction important for maintaining visual acuity.[23] It can occur in the setting of trauma, Graves ophthalmopathy, or orbital mass, among other causes. Reported cases in the literature do not include radiologic imaging, but clinical appearance is characteristic.

POSTERIOR SEGMENT INJURIES
Vitreous Hemorrhage

In the setting of trauma, orbital hemorrhage can accumulate within the posterior segment in multiple anatomic spaces. Blood accumulating in the vitreous is simply called vitreous hemorrhage

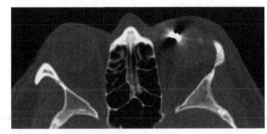

Fig. 11. Axial noncontrast CT of a patient with left medial scleral band used to treat retinal detachment mimicking foreign body. In the setting of trauma, eliciting a history of scleral banding may be crucial to differentiate from traumatic foreign body. Knowledge of the characteristic peripheral location can also aid in the correct diagnosis.

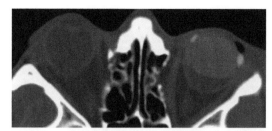

Fig. 12. Axial noncontrast CT. Silicone oil injected into the left vitreous, mimicking hemorrhage.

(Fig. 13). Hemorrhage can also collect in the space between the vitreous and retina. In addition, hemorrhage and fluid may seep into the potential spaces between the 3 layers of the globe, particularly when there has been laceration to 1 or more layers.

CHORIORETINAL INJURY

The retina is the innermost layer of the globe, and is securely attached to the choroid at its anterior margin, the ora serrata, and its posterior margin at the optic disc. The remainder is relatively loosely connected to the choroid. In the setting of trauma, a retinal tear can allow vitreous fluid and hemorrhage into the subretinal space. If the retina remains attached at the ora serrata and optic disc, hemorrhage lifting the retina off the choroid will have a characteristic V-shaped appearance on CT (Fig. 14).[9] If these attachments are also severed, the retina may become free-floating. The presence of subretinal hemorrhage in a child should raise suspicion for child abuse (Fig. 15). Nontraumatic causes of retinal detachment include inflammation and neoplasm.

Similarly, choroidal detachment occurs when hemorrhage or fluid collects in the suprachoroidal space between the choroid and sclera. The normal choroid extends from the ciliary body anteriorly to the optic nerve head posteriorly.

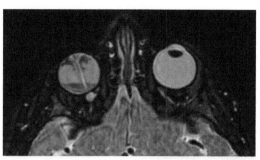

Fig. 14. Axial fat-suppressed T2-weighted image showing complete right retinal detachment with layering subretinal hemorrhage. This pediatric patient had primary hyperplastic vitreous with secondary retinal detachment; however the characteristic V-shaped detachment is illustrated.

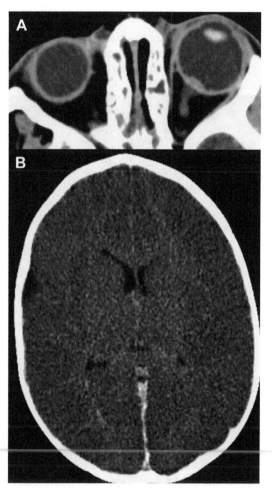

Fig. 15. (A) Axial noncontrast CT of a pediatric patient with left-sided subretinal hemorrhage. (B) Head CT of the same patient shows hemorrhage in the posterior horn of the right lateral ventricle in addition to posterior parafalcine subdural hemorrhage. The patient was later confirmed to be a victim of nonaccidental trauma.

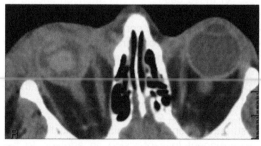

Fig. 13. Axial noncontrast CT of a patient with right-sided facial trauma shows right globe rupture evidenced by decreased globe volume and medial scleral discontinuity. There is prominent right vitreous hemorrhage.

Choroidal detachments occur in the setting of ocular hypotony, or decreased intraocular pressure. Trauma is one cause of ocular hypotony, which results in decreased pressure within the suprachoroidal space, allowing transudate to enter. If bridging arteries and veins between choroid and sclera are torn in the process, suprachoroidal hemorrhage can also occur. Suprachoroidal collections appear as biconvex, extending from the ciliary body anteriorly to the vortex veins posteriorly (Fig. 16).[9]

The morphology of hemorrhage can help distinguish the location in chorioretinal injury. Characteristically, choroidal detachment with suprachoroidal hemorrhage demonstrates a biconvex shape as opposed to a V-shaped configuration of retinal detachment and subretinal hemorrhage (Fig. 17).

Commotio Retinae

Commotio retinae, or Berlin edema, is a zonal area of retinal whitening caused by outer photoreceptor

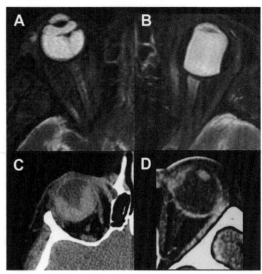

Fig. 17. Choroidal versus retinal hemorrhage. Axial fat-suppressed T2-weighted images (A, B) and axial noncontrast CT images (C, D) in 4 different patients. Characteristic V-shaped retinal detachment and hemorrhage is shown (A, C) in comparison with the biconvex shape of choroidal hemorrhage (B, D).

disruption and retinal pigment epithelial damage sustained by blunt trauma, often from assault, motor vehicle accident, or sports injury. It can result in loss of vision when affecting the macula.[24] Although there are no typical radiologic imaging findings, commotio retinae is often associated with preretinal, retinal, and subretinal hemorrhages and choroidal rupture, and, as such, a careful search for these findings should be made in this setting.[25]

PENETRATING OCULAR INJURIES

Penetrating ocular injuries can be obvious when large foreign bodies remain present (Fig. 18). However, they can be missed on physical examination if the injury is sealed off or if clinical signs are subtle.[26] In these cases, careful attention should be given to the detection of an intraorbital foreign body (IOFB), which is common, occurring in 1 of every 6 cases of orbital trauma.[27] Knowledge of the precise location and number of IOFBs is also important preoperatively. Extraocular IOFBs are typically managed conservatively, whereas those that are intraocular may require surgical intervention.[28] Sequelae of undetected IOFBs include posttraumatic endophthalmitis, potentially leading to permanent loss of vision, in addition to hyphema, cataract formation, vitreous hemorrhage, and retinal tears and detachment.[28] Failure to detect metallic foreign bodies on CT is potentially devastating if the patient goes on to MR imaging.

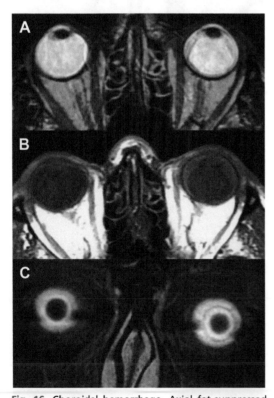

Fig. 16. Choroidal hemorrhage. Axial fat-suppressed T2-weighted (A), axial T1-weighted postcontrast (B), and coronal T2-weighted fat-suppressed (C) images of the orbits show biconvex collections in the left globe characteristic of suprachoroidal collections. The T2 signal is hypointense to vitreous and the T1 signal is intermediate, reflecting either hemorrhage or proteinaceous fluid.

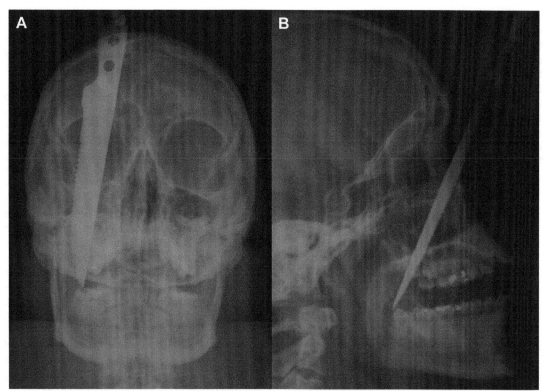

Fig. 18. (A) Anteroposterior and (B) lateral radiographs of a patient with transorbital penetrating knife injury extending through the maxillary sinus into the oral cavity.

CT is the gold standard for the detection of IOFBs,[27] with the ability to detect objects as small as 1 mm.[9] Metallic foreign bodies are well discerned on most CT window settings because of their high attenuation compared with the intraorbital soft tissues (Fig. 19B). MR imaging of a metallic IOFB demonstrates susceptibility artifact, which can limit evaluation of the orbit and surrounding soft tissues (see Fig. 19A).

Nonmetallic foreign bodies can present a diagnostic dilemma because they are less apparent on imaging. CT is more sensitive than MR imaging or ultrasonography for the detection of intraorbital glass. Sensitivity increases with increasing size (96% at 1.5 mm vs 48% at 0.5 mm), higher attenuation (range 80–550 HU), and anterior chamber location.[29] Wooden foreign bodies display a range of appearances on CT. Wood is a porous structure, and the relative amount of air and water within wood accounts for its attenuation on CT. For example, dry pine appears similarly to air on soft-tissue window settings (HU −656), whereas fresh pine, with greater water content, will appear at nearly water density on CT (HU −24).[27] A wooden foreign body can be difficult to identify when it mimics air, and should be scrutinized with wider window settings, especially in the

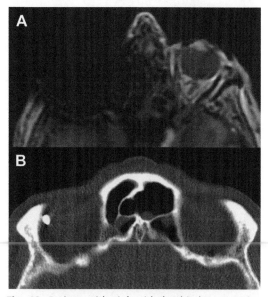

Fig. 19. Patient with right-sided orbital penetrating injury resulting in metallic foreign body. A magnetic resonance image (A) was first obtained without proper screening, showing significant susceptibility in the right orbit. Subsequent CT (B) shows the metallic foreign object in the right lateral orbit.

absence of fracture or if there are geometric margins (**Fig. 20**). The attenuation of wooden IOFBs has been shown to increase over time, a reported specific finding for wood; this likely results from body fluid displacing air within the porous foreign body.[30] Some advocate for MR imaging when CT is negative or equivocal in searching for a wood IOFB, because fat-suppressed postcontrast images can demonstrate surrounding inflammatory changes.[9]

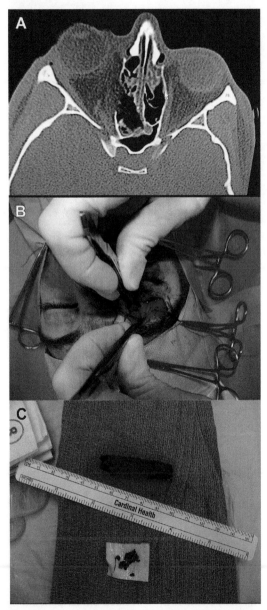

Fig. 20. Axial noncontrast CT (*A*) showing a hypodense foreign body traversing the orbit and right lamina papyracea into the ethmoid sinus. Intraoperative view (*B*) shows the deep penetrating injury and wooden foreign object that was removed (*C*).

CAROTID-CAVERNOUS FISTULAS

A carotid-cavernous fistula (CCF) forms when there is disruption of the wall of the cavernous internal carotid artery (ICA), resulting in arteriovenous shunting from the ICA into the cavernous sinus. Although CCF in most cases is not secondary to orbital trauma, it can result in multiple orbit-related findings, and therefore is an important entity to consider in posttraumatic orbital imaging. The typical mechanism for a posttraumatic CCF involves a skull-base fracture extending through the sphenoid bone and bony carotid canal, or penetrating injury to the posterior orbit or cavernous sinus.[31] When arterialized flow develops in the cavernous sinus, increased venous pressure can lead to flow reversal in the veins draining into the cavernous sinus, including the ophthalmic veins. If untreated, a progressive increase in intraocular pressure can ultimately cause retinal hypoperfusion and retinal ischemia. Ocular symptoms, including ocular chemosis, proptosis, glaucoma, and visual loss, typically do not present immediately but rather days or weeks after the initial trauma.[31] Pulsating exophthalmos and objective pulsatile tinnitus are also occasionally seen along with deficits of cranial nerves III through VI.[9]

Imaging of the head and orbits is valuable in the diagnosis of CCF. Typically CT or MR imaging demonstrates dilation of the superior ophthalmic vein, proptosis, and extraocular muscle enlargement, all findings potentially demonstrable on noncontrast studies.[9] Contrast-enhanced CT or MR imaging can provide additional diagnostic clues, including illustration of cavernous sinus distension and improved visualization of ophthalmic vein enlargement (**Fig. 21**). Definitive diagnosis requires digital subtraction angiography (DSA), which shows early aberrant filling of the cavernous sinus and dilated veins leading away from the sinus, including the superior and inferior ophthalmic veins and the superior and inferior petrosal sinuses. DSA can also provide access for endovascular therapy for CCF, with treatment options including detachable balloon embolization, transvenous embolization, or covered-stent repair of ICA laceration.[32]

OPTIC NERVE INJURY

Traumatic optic neuropathy (TON) is a rare but important potential result of head trauma, with recent estimates suggesting that optic nerve injury occurs in approximately 0.5% to 5% of all closed head injuries and up to 10% of patients with craniofacial fractures.[33] TON can be subdivided into 2 main types, direct or indirect, defined by mechanism of injury to the optic nerve.[34] Direct TON

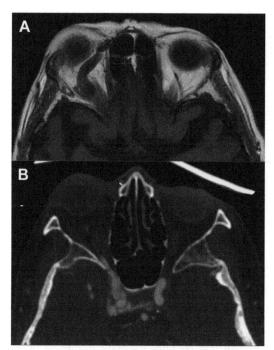

Fig. 21. (*A*) Axial T1-weighted image shows right-sided proptosis and marked dilatation of the right superior ophthalmic vein in this patient after direct facial trauma. (*B*) Axial CT angiography shows an abnormal enlargement of the right cavernous sinus with a convex lateral border. Note the abnormal early venous enhancement in the right side of the cavernous sinus, consistent with arteriovenous shunting in this patient with a direct posttraumatic carotid-cavernous fistula.

occurs when the optic nerve is damaged by a transorbital penetrating injury such as from a bullet or knife. Indirect TON includes all other nonpenetrating sequelae of trauma, including mass effect from retrobulbar hemorrhage and deceleration injuries that subject the optic nerve to violent rotatory forces. Such indirect mechanisms of injury may compress or tear the optic nerve or its associated vascular supply. TON typically produces clinical findings common to most optic neuropathies, including decreased visual acuity, color, and visual field, with visual acuity often 20/400 or less on the affected side.[33] Patients with TON often have severe injuries requiring immediate attention; the diagnosis of TON may be delayed until a detailed visual assessment can be performed.

In patients with facial trauma and subsequent decrease in visual acuity, neuroimaging is used to evaluate for potential causes of TON. In particular, noncontrast CT through the orbits is valuable in the assessment of any fracture involving the orbital apex that could compromise the optic nerve (**Fig. 22**).[33] In cases of TON related to a

retrobulbar hemorrhage, noncontrast CT will allow for the characterization of the volume and extent of hemorrhage in the orbit, potentially guiding surgical decompression (**Fig. 23**). In situations where a trauma patient is clinically stable and able to tolerate MR imaging, direct visualization of the optic nerve can reveal abnormal hyperintensity in the nerve on T2-weighted images. In cases of posttraumatic compromise of the vascular supply to the optic nerve, diffusion-weighted imaging can demonstrate reduced diffusivity in the optic nerve, suggesting ischemic injury (see **Fig. 22**B, C). The ability to integrate detailed multisequence MR imaging of the orbits, however, is often unfeasible, despite its advantage in the demonstration of soft-tissue abnormality.

In patients sustaining traumatic injury to the optic nerves, the main treatment options remain close observation, high-dose corticosteroid therapy, surgical decompression, or a combination thereof.[33] However, given the lack of large observational studies or randomized controlled trials assessing patient outcomes after treatment of TON, the optimal treatment algorithm remains controversial. Future treatments currently being investigated include neuroprotective drugs and other therapies to enhance visual recovery following trauma.[33]

Diagnostic checklist orbital CT

ACD: Ensure the ACD is symmetric bilaterally. Corneal laceration, globe rupture, and lens dislocation will result in ACD asymmetry.

Lens density: A traumatic cataract will manifest with unilateral lens hypodensity.

Lens position: Careful attention should be paid to lens position. Complete dislocation is most common posteriorly into the vitreous. Partial dislocation may show subtle asymmetry away from the side of zonule fiber disruption.

Globe shape: The globe should demonstrate a smooth contour. Globe rupture may show focal discontinuity. Staphylomas have a characteristic location and morphology.

Foreign body: IOFB is an operative emergency and should be reported immediately. Metallic foreign bodies are usually conspicuous on CT and preclude MR imaging. Wood or other hypodense organic foreign bodies can be subtle.

Posterior segment density: Vitreous, retinal, and choroidal hemorrhage each have a characteristic location and configuration.

Fracture: Careful attention should be paid to the osseous structures surrounding the orbit, which are commonly fractured in facial trauma.

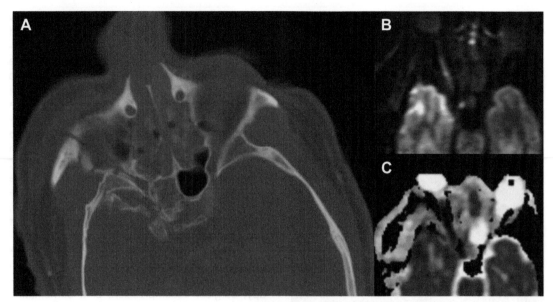

Fig. 22. A patient with right-sided visual loss after facial trauma. (*A*) Axial CT shows a complex orbital fracture with a bony fracture fragment from the right orbital apex situated within the optic canal. Axial diffusion-weighted imaging (*B*) and apparent diffusion coefficient map (*C*) show diffusion restriction with the intracanalicular and orbital segments of the right optic nerve, a finding that confirms traumatic disruption of the vascular supply to the optic nerve and resultant nerve ischemia. Right anterior temporal traumatic injury is also present.

ACKNOWLEDGMENTS

The authors would like to acknowledge Dr Kristine Mosier for her case contributions.

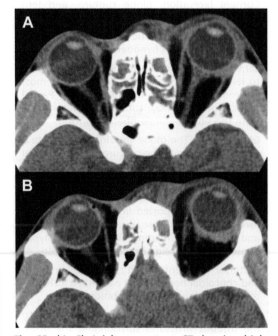

Fig. 23. (*A*, *B*) Axial noncontrast CT showing high-density left orbital retrobulbar hemorrhage.

REFERENCES

1. Lee HJ, Jilani M, Frohman L, et al. CT of orbital trauma. Emerg Radiol 2004;10(4):168–72.
2. Harlan JB Jr, Pieramici DJ. Evaluation of patients with ocular trauma. Ophthalmol Clin North Am 2002;15(2):153–61.
3. Iinuma T, Hirota Y, Ishio K. Orbital wall fractures. Conventional views and CT. Rhinology 1994;32(2):81–3.
4. Joseph JM, Glavas IP. Orbital fractures: a review. Clin Ophthalmol 2011;5:95–100.
5. Rhea JT, Rao PM, Novelline RA. Helical CT and three-dimensional CT of facial and orbital injury. Radiol Clin North Am 1999;37(3):489–513.
6. Joseph DP, Pieramici DJ, Beauchamp NJ Jr. Computed tomography in the diagnosis and prognosis of open-globe injuries. Ophthalmology 2000; 107(10):1899–906.
7. Wang JW, Tang C, Pan BR. Data analysis of low dose multislice helical CT scan in orbital trauma. Int J Ophthalmol 2012;5(3):366–9. http://dx.doi.org/10.3980/j.issn.2222-3959.2012.03.22.
8. Bord SP, Linden J. Trauma to the globe and orbit. Emerg Med Clin North Am 2008;26(1):97–123,. vi–vii.

9. Kubal WS. Imaging of orbital trauma. Radiographics 2008;28(6):1729–39.

10. Jank S, Emshoff R, Etzelsdorfer M, et al. Ultrasound versus computed tomography in the imaging of orbital floor fractures. J Oral Maxillofac Surg 2004; 62(2):150–4.

11. Kim SY, Lee JH, Lee YJ, et al. Diagnostic value of the anterior chamber depth of a globe on CT for detecting open-globe injury. Eur Radiol 2010;20(5):1079–84.

12. Caranci F, Cicala D, Cappabianca S, et al. Orbital fractures: role of imaging. Semin Ultrasound CT MR 2012;33(5):385–91.

13. Brandt MT, Haug RH. Traumatic hyphema: a comprehensive review. J Oral Maxillofac Surg 2001;59(12): 1462–70.

14. De Leon-Ortega JE, Girkin CA. Ocular trauma-related glaucoma. Ophthalmol Clin North Am 2002; 15(2):215–23.

15. Netland KE, Martinez J, LaCour OJ 3rd, et al. Traumatic anterior lens dislocation: a case report. J Emerg Med 1999;17(4):637–9.

16. Dunkin JM, Crum AV, Swanger RS, et al. Globe trauma. Semin Ultrasound CT MR 2011;32(1):51–6.

17. Segev Y, Goldstein M, Lazar M, et al. CT appearance of a traumatic cataract. AJNR Am J Neuroradiol 1995;16(5):1174–5.

18. Gupta A, Rahman I, Leatherbarrow B. Open globe injuries in children: factors predictive of a poor final visual acuity. Eye (Lond) 2009;23(3): 621–5.

19. Arey ML, Mootha VV, Whittemore AR, et al. Computed tomography in the diagnosis of occult open-globe injuries. Ophthalmology 2007;114(8): 1448–52.

20. Hoffstetter P, Schreyer AG, Schreyer CI, et al. (MD-CT) in the diagnosis of uncertain open globe injuries. Rofo 2010;182(2):151–4.

21. Weissman JL, Beatty RL, Hirsch WL, et al. Enlarged anterior chamber: CT finding of a ruptured globe. AJNR Am J Neuroradiol 1995; 16(Suppl 4):936–8.

22. Swanger RS, Crum AV, Klett ZG, et al. Postsurgical imaging of the globe. Semin Ultrasound CT MR 2011;32(1):57–63.

23. Love JN, Bertram-Love NE. Luxation of the globe. Am J Emerg Med 1993;11(1):61–3.

24. Blanch RJ, Good PA, Shah P, et al. Visual outcomes after blunt ocular trauma. Ophthalmology 2013; 120(8):1588–91.

25. Youssri AI, Young LH. Closed-globe contusion injuries of the posterior segment. Int Ophthalmol Clin 2002;42(3):79–86.

26. Khaw PT, Shah P, Elkington AR. Injury to the eye. BMJ 2004;328(7430):36–8.

27. Adesanya OO, Dawkins DM. Intraorbital wooden foreign body (IOFB): mimicking air on CT. Emerg Radiol 2007;14(1):45–9.

28. Pinto A, Brunese L, Daniele S, et al. Role of computed tomography in the assessment of intraorbital foreign bodies. Semin Ultrasound CT MR 2012; 33(5):392–5.

29. Gor DM, Kirsch CF, Leen J, et al. Radiologic differentiation of intraocular glass: evaluation of imaging techniques, glass types, size, and effect of intraocular hemorrhage. AJR Am J Roentgenol 2001; 177(5):1199–203.

30. Yamashita K, Noguchi T, Mihara F, et al. An intraorbital wooden foreign body: description of a case and a variety of CT appearances. Emerg Radiol 2007; 14(1):41–3.

31. Provenzale J. CT and MR imaging of acute cranial trauma. Emerg Radiol 2007;14(1):1–12.

32. Ng PP, Higashida RT, Cullen S, et al. Endovascular strategies for carotid cavernous and intracerebral dural arteriovenous fistulas. Neurosurg Focus 2003;15(4):ECP1.

33. Warner N, Eggenberger E. Traumatic optic neuropathy: a review of the current literature. Curr Opin Ophthalmol 2010;21(6):459–62.

34. Steinsapir KD, Goldberg RA. Traumatic optic neuropathy: an evolving understanding. Am J Ophthalmol 2011;151(6):928–33.

Skull Base Fractures and Their Complications

Kristen L. Baugnon, MD*, Patricia A. Hudgins, MD

KEYWORDS

- Skull base trauma • CSF leak • Basilar skull fracture • CSF rhinorrhea

KEY POINTS

- Skull base fractures are managed based on associated intracranial injury and complications, including vascular and cranial nerve injury and cerebrospinal fluid (CSF) leak.
- Anterior cranial fossa fractures, particularly comminuted and oblique frontobasal fractures, are commonly associated with CSF leak, either acute or delayed in presentation.
- Transverse middle cranial fossa fractures extending through the carotid canal are at increased risk for vascular injury, and should prompt screening with vascular studies, such as CT angiography.
- Thin-section multiplanar CT reformations, as well as 3-dimensional reconstructions, are helpful in the detection of subtle skull base fractures.

INTRODUCTION

Head trauma is one of the most common reasons for visits to the emergency department in the United States. According to the 2013 National Trauma Data Bank maintained by the American College of Surgeons, of 833,311 adult trauma admissions reported from 805 facilities across the United States, approximately 36% sustained an injury to the head.[1] Skull base fractures, those fractures that extend through the floor of the anterior, middle, or posterior cranial fossa, occur in an estimated 7% to 16% of nonpenetrating head injuries, and are due to a relatively high-velocity trauma, most often high-speed motor vehicle accidents, although motorcycle collisions, pedestrian injuries, falls, and assault are additional associated causes.[2] Penetrating trauma, particularly gunshot wounds, are seen much less frequently, accounting for less than 10% of cases.[3]

Skull base injury is often seen in the setting of complex facial or orbital fractures, and detection of basilar skull fractures is important, as even linear nondisplaced fractures can be associated with numerous critical complications, including intracranial and orbital injuries, cerebrospinal fluid (CSF) leak, cranial nerve palsies, and vascular injuries. Although facial fractures often require repair to improve function and cosmesis, the management of patients with skull base injury is dependent on the extent of associated intracranial injury and other complications. The associated risk and extent of complications often depends on the location and pattern of the fracture, which is in turn determined by the mechanism of injury and type of impact.

NORMAL ANATOMY

The skull base is made up of 7 bones, the paired frontal and temporal bones, and the unpaired ethmoid, sphenoid, and occipital bones. It is divided into anterior, central, and posterior regions, which form the floor of the anterior, middle, and posterior cranial fossae.

The anterior skull base, formed by the frontal and ethmoid bones, separates the anterior and inferior frontal lobes and olfactory structures within

Disclosures: Dr P.A. Hudgins is an author, contributor, and shareholder for Amirsys, Inc.
Department of Radiology and Imaging Sciences, Emory University School of Medicine, 1364 Clifton Road, Atlanta, GA 30322, USA
* Corresponding author.
E-mail address: kmlloyd@emory.edu

Neuroimag Clin N Am 24 (2014) 439–465
http://dx.doi.org/10.1016/j.nic.2014.03.001
1052-5149/14/$ – see front matter © 2014 Elsevier Inc. All rights reserved.

neuroimaging.theclinics.com

the anterior cranial fossa from the orbits and the sinonasal cavity. The lateral and anterior borders of the anterior cranial fossa are formed by the orbital plate of the frontal bone and the posterior table of the frontal sinus. Inferiorly, the floor of the anterior cranial fossa is formed by the cribriform plates and roof of the ethmoid sinuses. The posterior border between the anterior and central skull base is formed by the lesser wing of the sphenoid bone, including the clinoid process, and the planum sphenoidale (Fig. 1).

Deep clefts lateral to the midline crista galli form the olfactory grooves, which house the olfactory bulbs. The floor of the olfactory groove is formed by the cribriform plates, which are inherently thin, with multiple small foramina through which the small branches of the olfactory nerve pass. The lateral lamella is a thin bone connecting the cribriform plate with the fovea ethmoidalis, or the roof of the ethmoid sinuses, all part of the ethmoid bone. In addition to the cribriform plate foramina, the anterior skull base contains the anterior and posterior ethmoid artery foramina, which should not be confused with fractures; these may represent significant sources of epistaxis, if injured (Fig. 2).

The central skull base, formed by the sphenoid and anterior temporal bones, separates the pituitary gland (within the sella), the cavernous sinuses (including the carotid artery and cranial nerves), the Meckel cave, and the temporal lobes superiorly from the sphenoid sinus anteriorly and inferiorly, and the extracranial soft tissues deep to the skull base inferiorly, including the masticator, parotid, parapharyngeal, and pharyngeal mucosal spaces. The anterior border of the central skull base is formed by the posterior margin of the lesser wing of the sphenoid bone, clinoid process and tuberculum sella. The floor is formed by the greater wing and central body of the sphenoid bone, the sphenoid sinus, and the sella. The posterior border between the central and posterior skull base is formed by the superior margin of the petrous ridge of the temporal bone, the basi sphenoid portion of the clivus, and the dorsum sella (see Fig. 1). In addition to housing the pituitary gland, the central skull base contains numerous foramina and canals through which many important structures pass, including cranial nerves (CNs) II to VI and the internal carotid artery (Fig. 3, Table 1).

The posterior skull base is formed by the posterior temporal bone and the occipital bone, and separates the posterior fossa structures, including the cerebellum and brainstem, from the extracranial soft tissues: the posterior nasopharynx, retropharyngeal space, carotid space, and perivertebral space. The anterior border is formed by the petrous ridge of the temporal bone superiorly, and the clivus (basi occiput portion) inferiorly. The inferior border includes the occipital condyles and the mastoid portion of the temporal bone, and the posterior skull base extends posteriorly to the squamous portion of the occipital bone (see Fig. 1). Some consider the temporal bone proper to be the lateral, or posterolateral skull base.

The largest foramen of the skull base, foramen magnum, is located within the posterior skull base, and transmits the medulla oblongata (cervicomedullary junction), vertebral arteries, and spinal portion of CN XI. Other major foramina within the posterior skull base include the internal auditory canal (CN VII, VIII, and labyrinthine artery), jugular foramen (pars nervosa anteriorly: CN IX, inferior petrosal sinus, and Jacobsen nerve; pars vascularis posteriorly: CN X, XI, Arnolds nerve and jugular bulb), and hypoglossal canal (CN XII) (Figs. 4 and 5).

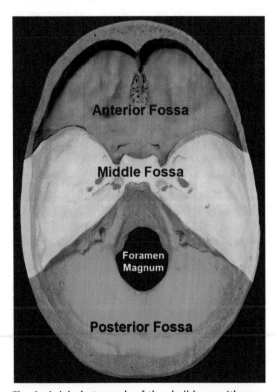

Fig. 1. Axial photograph of the skull base with overlays demonstrating the anterior, middle, and posterior cranial fossae. (*Courtesy of* Kevin Makowski and Eric Jablonowski, Emory University, Atlanta, GA.)

PATHOLOGY

Fractures through the skull base are often the sequelae of high-velocity impact and may be linear

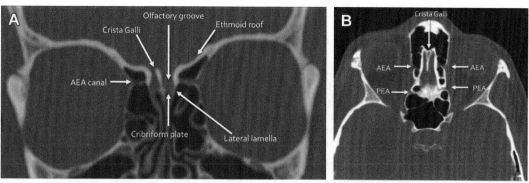

Fig. 2. Anterior skull base. (*A*) Coronal CT demonstrating the olfactory groove, bordered by the crista galli, cribriform plate, and lateral lamella. The lateral lamella extends cranially to form the ethmoid roof. Note the horizontal trajectory of the anterior ethmoid artery canal, with its corticated margins and medial tapering. (*B*) Axial CT showing bilateral anterior and posterior ethmoid artery canals (AEA and PEA respectively), corticated and in a characteristic location that should not be mistaken for fracture.

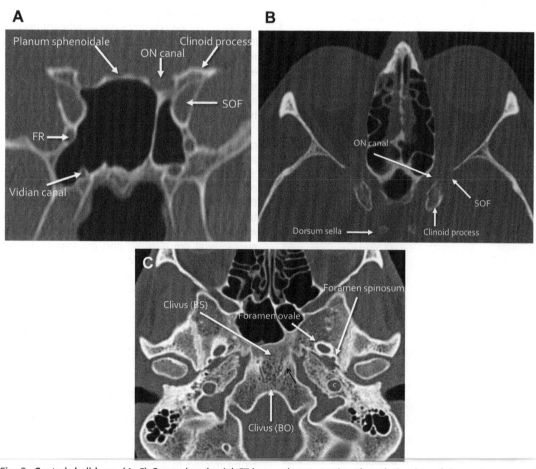

Fig. 3. Central skull base. (*A, B*) Coronal and axial CT image demonstrating the relationship of the optic nerve and superior orbital fissure to the clinoid process, with the optic nerve medial to the clinoid process, and the superior orbital fissure inferior and lateral to the clinoid process. Note the planum sphenoidale, foramen rotundum (FR) transmitting V2 along the lateral sphenoid sinus, and vidian canal transmitting the vidian nerve inferomedially. (*C*) Axial CT through the middle cranial fossa floor showing the "high-heel shoe" appearance of foramen ovale (the "toe of the shoeprint"), and foramen spinosum (the "heel") within the sphenoid bone. The carotid canal ("c") enters the petrous portion of the temporal bone, extending cranially with vertical and horizontal segments. The basisphenoid (BS) portion of the clivus superiorly and anteriorly is located within the middle cranial fossa, whereas the basi occiput (BO) portion of the clivus is a portion of the occipital bone, within the posterior cranial fossa. Note the sclerotic fused sphenooccipital synchondrosis/fissure (*thin black arrow*). ON, optic nerve; SOF, superior orbital fissure.

Table 1
Central skull base foramina and their contents

Foramen	Contents
Optic nerve canal	CN II (optic nerve) Ophthalmic artery
Superior orbital fissure	CN III (oculomotor nerve) CN IV (trochlear nerve) CN V1 (ophthalmic branch of the trigeminal nerve) CN VI (abducens nerve) Superior ophthalmic vein
Foramen rotundum	CN V2 (maxillary branch of trigeminal nerve)
Foramen ovale	CN V3 (mandibular branch of trigeminal nerve)
Carotid canal	Internal carotid artery Sympathetic plexus
Foramen spinosum	Middle meningeal artery
Vidian canal	Vidian nerve and artery
Foramen lacerum	Cartilage

Abbreviation: CN, cranial nerve.

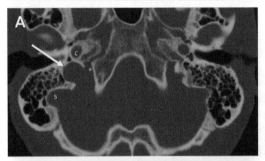

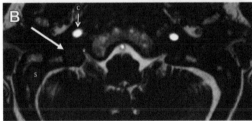

Fig. 4. Posterior cranial fossa and skull base. (*A, B*) CT and MRI images showing the sigmoid sinus (s) as it extends caudally toward the jugular foramen (*arrow*), with the dominant pars vascularis posteriorly and the pars nervosa (*asterisk*) anteromedially. The pars nervosa contains the inferior petrosal sinus and glossopharyngeal nerve (seen on T2-weighted MRI). Note the proximity of the jugular foramen to the carotid canal (c).

or comminuted, with a potentially complex imaging appearance. Fracture patterns and associated complications depend on the location of the injury, which is often determined by the mechanism of injury and type of impact. Table 2 outlines the most commonly encountered complications associated with site of injury.

Anterior Skull Base Fractures

Classification/Etiology

Direct frontal trauma often results in anterior skull base fractures, so-called frontobasal injuries, with the "frontal" component of fractures involving the upper facial third (frontal bone/sinus and superior orbital rim), and "basal" component of fracture involving the anterior skull base (cribriform plate, ethmoid roofs, and planum sphenoidale). Numerous classification systems for frontobasal injuries have been described in an attempt to stratify complications and guide management. One of the more recent anatomic classification systems evolved based on cadaveric studies demonstrating unique reproducible fracture patterns, similar to Lefort facial fractures, and classifies frontobasal fractures into types I through III.[4,5]

Type I frontobasal fractures are generally associated with a relatively lower impact frontal injury, and are defined as linear fractures that initially parallel the cribriform plate, then may extend posteriorly along the sella and petrous ridge to separate the anterior and middle cranial fossa from the posterior cranial fossa. These generally are more medially located, involving the medial third of the supraorbital rim (Fig. 6), and are less frequently associated with complications. Type II fractures are composed of more lateral vertical linear fractures of the frontal calvarium and anterior skull base and often extend to involve the lateral two-thirds of the supraorbital rim, the squamous portion of the temporal bone, the orbital roof, the lateral orbital wall, or the orbital apex. These are more frequently associated with CSF leak and intracranial injury (Fig. 7). Finally, type III fractures combine central and lateral frontobasilar fractures, often with comminution of the entire frontal bone, orbital roof, and lateral cranial vault (Fig. 8). Type II and III fractures are more frequently associated with concomitant midface injuries and are thought to be related to a higher-velocity impact from a lateral or inferior frontal or supraorbital vector. As one might suspect, because type III fractures are associated with the greatest force, they are most often associated with complications such as intracranial injury and CSF leak, reportedly in up to 25% of cases.[5]

One additional classification system, devised by Piccirilli and colleagues,[6] divides frontobasal

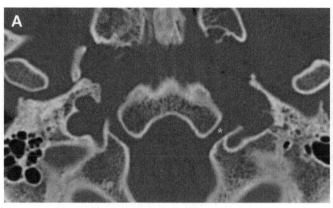
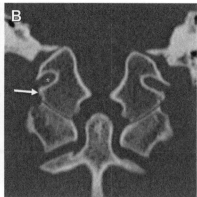

Fig. 5. Posterior cranial fossa. (*A*, *B*) Axial and coronal CT images showing the hypoglossal canal (*asterisk*) in relation to the occipital condyle (*arrow*).

fractures into types A to C, each denoting a different surgical approach for management. Type A fractures involve only the anterior table of the frontal sinus, whereas type B fractures involve the posterior table (**Fig. 9**). Type C fractures include any frontobasal injury that does not involve the frontal sinus. Fractures extending through the posterior table of the frontal sinus (type B), particularly when comminuted, in addition to potentially causing CSF leak, can ultimately result in the development of a mucocele, due to entrapped mucosa along the fracture line. Thus, these fractures may require a different surgical approach, including frontal sinus obliteration (removing the mucosa and filling the sinus with fat or other materials, such as hydroxyapatite) or cranialization (removal of the posterior table mucosa and bone, and performing any duraplasty needed at the time). Both of these surgeries should involve surgical obstruction of the outflow tracts.[7] Some

investigators currently advocate cranialization if the fracture involves more than 25% of the posterior table of the frontal sinus.[8] Less displaced fractures can be managed conservatively, or via endoscopic approaches.[8,9]

Complications
The management of skull base fractures is based on anticipated potential complications. Although many facial fractures may require repair to maintain function and cosmesis, skull base fractures often require repair only if there is associated intracranial injury requiring decompression, persistent CSF leak, or significant cranial nerve or vascular injury. Also, extensive fractures through the posterior table of the frontal sinus may require surgical repair to prevent mucocele formation. Anterior skull base injuries are frequently seen in conjunction with frontal lobe contusions and intraorbital injuries, which are discussed in the article by

Table 2
Location of skull base fracture and frequently associated complications

Location	Complication
Anterior skull base	Intraorbital injury Sinonasal CSF leak/meningoencephalocele Anosmia (CN I injury)
Central skull base	Vascular injury (ICA occlusion, dissection, pseudoaneurysm, aneurysm, CCF) Cranial nerve injury (optic nerve, CN III, IV, V, and VI) Horner syndrome
Posterolateral skull base (temporal bone)	Vascular injury (ICA) CN VII or VIII injury Mastoid CSF leak/meningoencephalocele
Posterior skull base	Venous vascular injury or vertebrobasilar injury Lower cranial nerve injuries (CN IX, X, XII, or XII) Craniocervical junction and cervical spine injuries

Abbreviations: CCF, carotid cavernous fistula; CN, cranial nerve; CSF, cerebrospinal fluid; ICA, internal carotid artery.

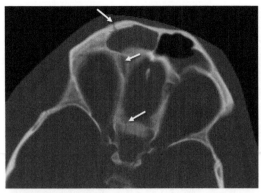

Fig. 6. Type I frontobasal fracture. Axial CT demonstrating a linear fracture through the anterior cranial fossa medially (*arrows*), traversing the anterior and posterior table of the frontal sinus, paralleling the cribriform plate, then extending through the planum sphenoidale.

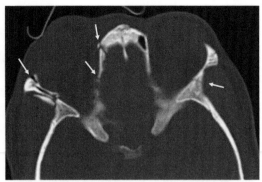

Fig. 8. Type III frontobasal fracture. Axial CT image demonstrating a comminuted and displaced transversely oriented anterior skull base fracture (*arrows*) extending across the orbital roofs and ethmoid roofs, with involvement of the lateral orbital walls. Given the comminution and medial and lateral anterior skull base involvement, this is a type III frontobasal fracture. Note pneumocephalus and orbital and soft tissue emphysema.

Gupta and colleagues, elsewhere in this issue. The most commonly associated complications are CSF leak (with or without meningitis), and injury to the olfactory nerve, resulting in anosmia; these are unique to the anterior skull base.

CSF leak after trauma occurs when there is both an osseous defect and a tear of the closely adherent dura, leading to egress of CSF from the subarachnoid space into the sinonasal cavity (in the setting of frontobasal fractures) or into the middle ear cavity and mastoid air cells (in the setting of temporal bone trauma). CSF rhinorrhea or otorrhea is the usual clinical presentation. There are rare reports, in the setting of complex orbital roof injuries, of oculorrhea and intermittent periorbital swelling and tearing due to accumulation of CSF.[10] The more comminuted and displaced fractures, such as type III frontobasal fractures, carry

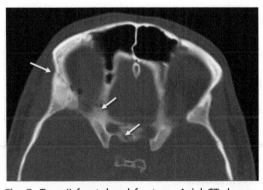

Fig. 7. Type II frontobasal fracture. Axial CT demonstrating a linear fracture through the lateral aspect of the anterior cranial fossa (*arrows*), traversing the orbital roof, and extending along the optic nerve canal to the tuberculum sella posteriorly.

the greatest risk of CSF leak. Communication with the flora of the nasal or middle ear cavities results in meningitis, reportedly in up to 50% of cases, if the leak is not repaired.[11] The risk is approximately 1% in the first 24 hours, increasing to 18% at the end of 2 weeks (**Fig. 10**).[12,13] In fact, any patient presenting clinically with recurrent episodes of meningitis (particularly in the setting of prior trauma) should be evaluated for occult CSF fistula.[12]

Traumatic CSF leak, which is the most common form of CSF leak, occurs in 10% to 30% of skull base fractures, and most often presents as CSF rhinorrhea (in 80% of cases).[2,14,15] Eighty percent of cases will present in the first 48 hours after injury, and most (up to 95%) will present with CSF rhinorrhea in the first 3 months after trauma. The delay in symptom onset is primarily due to resolution of the initial posttraumatic edema and hemorrhage, combined with increased mobility as the patient progresses through rehabilitation. However, a small minority of patients (5%) will present in a more delayed fashion, months to even decades after their trauma, possibly due to fracture fragments slowly eroding and thinning the dura over time (**Fig. 11**).[16]

Most posttraumatic CSF leaks, up to 85%, are acute in presentation, and heal spontaneously with conservative management such as bed rest, head elevation, and stool softeners.[17–19] Occasionally patients will require CSF diversion with lumbar drain or external ventricular drain placement if the leaks do not resolve in approximately 2 to 7 days.[12,18] One recent study demonstrated good results in high-risk patients with the

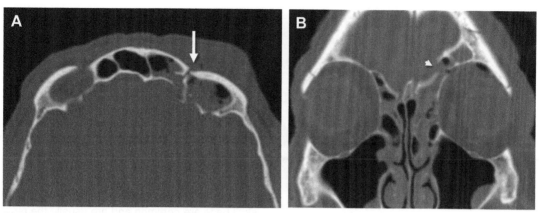

Fig. 9. Axial (A) and coronal (B) CT images of a comminuted and displaced frontobasal fracture with extension through both anterior (arrow) and posterior (arrowhead) tables of the frontal sinus and orbital roof, with intraorbital hematoma and emphysema.

administration of acetazolamide in the early post-traumatic period.[20] Of course patients presenting with acute CSF rhinorrhea with intracranial pathology requiring immediate surgical treatment, such as frontal lobe hematomas or depressed skull fractures, will undergo open intracranial repair of fractures and duraplasty at the time of the surgery. Those with persistent leaks for longer than 7 to 10 days, in spite of CSF diversion, often require repair, either intracranial or endoscopic. Larger skull base defects (>1.5 cm) or severely comminuted fractures, particularly if a meningoencephalocele is present, are associated with a worse prognosis for spontaneous resolution, and will require surgical repair.[12,21,22] The use of prophylactic antibiotics to avoid meningitis is a controversial topic. A recent large meta-analysis reviewing the outcomes of 1241 patients showed overall no statistically significant decrease in meningitis in patients treated with prophylactic antibiotics.[23] Similarly, a Cochrane review of 2168 patients in 2011 showed no evidence to support the use of prophylactic antibiotics, but recommended the need for large randomized controlled trials in the future.[14]

Loss of smell, or anosmia, as a result of olfactory nerve injury, is a relatively common complication

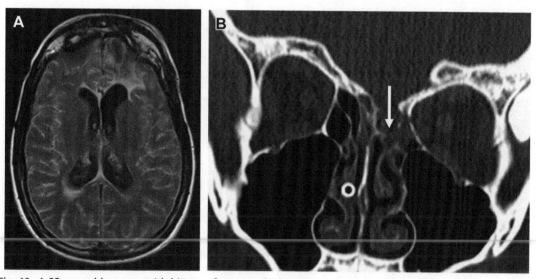

Fig. 10. A 32-year-old woman with history of motor vehicle accident 9 years previously, presented with CSF rhinorrhea, altered mental status and seizure. (A) Axial FLAIR image shows encephalomalacia in the anterior and inferior left frontal lobe, adjacent to the left frontal bone deformity from prior depressed skull fracture. Note nonsuppression of CSF signal in the sulci and ventricles compatible with meningitis and ventriculitis; there was growth of gram-positive cocci on lumbar puncture. (B) Coronal reformat CT shows a large left lateral lamella and ethmoid roof defect (arrow), with polypoid nondependent soft tissue adjacent to the dehiscence, compatible with a posttraumatic meningoencephalocele, the source of the CSF leak.

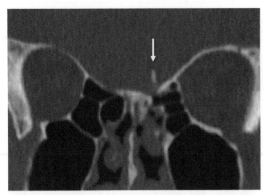

Fig. 11. A 73-year-old man with persistent rhinorrhea since trauma 6 months previously, positive for beta 2 transferrin. Coronal CT image demonstrates a focal defect within the left ethmoid roof with an adjacent vertically oriented fracture fragment (*arrow*), likely the source of dural tear.

after trauma, with an overall incidence of up to 7%, and an increased risk in anterior skull base fractures, particularly medial fractures along the cribriform plates. Traumatic CSF leak, particularly when repair is required, has been associated with an increased risk of anosmia as well. Only

approximately 10% of all patients with traumatic anosmia are estimated to recover sense of smell, often in a delayed fashion, months to years after the injury.[24]

Central Skull Base Fractures

Classification/Etiology

Extension of frontobasal fractures from frontal impact can occur in a sagittal or oblique fashion through the central skull base with involvement of the sella and sphenoid sinus, and, in some cases, the temporal bone (Fig. 12). Transverse fractures in a coronal plane through the central skull base are common and are usually the result of high velocity lateral impact to the lateral frontal bone, zygoma, temporal, or parietal bone. Several transverse fracture patterns have been described, including transverse or oblique/diagonal patterns; these are related to the mechanism of injury. Transverse fractures extend through the sphenoid sinus, either anteriorly or posteriorly, depending on type of impact, and can propagate laterally through the greater sphenoid wing and squamosal temporal bones, or be associated with temporal bone fractures (Fig. 13). The more anterior

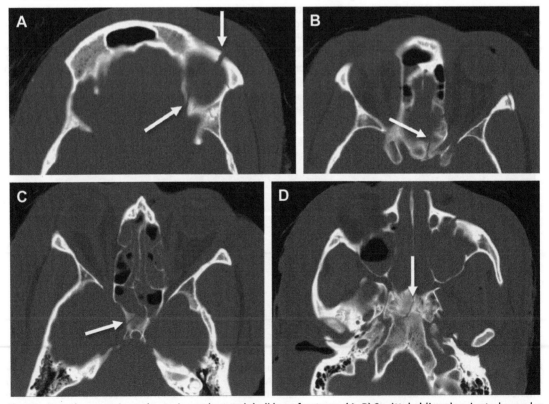

Fig. 12. Complex comminuted anterior and central skull base fractures. (*A–D*) Sagittal obliquely oriented complex comminuted left frontobasal fracture (*arrows*) extending along the supraorbital rim and orbital roof (*A*), along the left ethmoid roof and planum sphenoidale (*B*), through the sphenoid sinus walls (*C*), and into the basi sphenoid portion of the clivus (*C, D*).

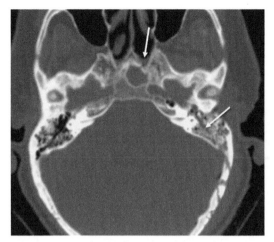

Fig. 13. Longitudinal left temporal bone fracture extends medially to involve the sphenoid sinus walls (*arrows*).

transverse fractures often involve the posterior aspect of the anterior cranial fossa (posterior ethmoid roof) and may extend through the clinoid processes, involving both the orbital apex and the superior orbital fissures and potentially resulting in cranial nerve or vascular injuries. The more posterior transverse patterns may involve the temporal bones bilaterally, extending along the sphenopetrosal synchondrosis, with involvement of the posterior sphenoid sinus and/or clivus (**Fig. 14**). Oblique central skull base fractures, often associated with facial fractures and type II or III frontobasal fractures, are more often associated with CSF leak. Transverse fractures are more commonly associated with vascular and cranial nerve injuries, although these can be seen in both types of central skull base fractures, depending on their course.[25,26]

Involvement of the clivus with central and posterior skull base fractures deserves special mention. These fractures are rare, accounting for about 2% of all cranial fractures, but are associated with high mortality (24%–80%) because of location and proximity to the brainstem, as well as high incidence of neurologic and vascular injury (up to 46%).[27] There are 2 characteristic patterns of clival injury: transverse or oblique, and longitudinal.[27,28] Transverse or oblique fractures, similar to other transverse central skull base fractures, are caused by a lateral or crushing injury, and are commonly associated with cranial nerve and internal carotid artery (ICA) injury (**Fig. 15**). Conversely, longitudinal clival fractures are more complex, are due to axial loading mechanism from the vertex, and are often associated with vertebrobasilar injury and brainstem infarction.[29] Longitudinal clival fractures are seen in conjunction with craniocervical junction injuries, and retroclival hematomas. A hallmark of clival fracture clinically is the presence of sixth nerve palsy, due to the location of the Dorello canal within the clivus.[30] Other cranial nerve injuries are also frequently seen.[27,28]

Complications

Central skull base fractures are primarily managed based on associated complications. Many are associated with intracranial injuries, including multicompartmental hemorrhage, temporal lobe parenchymal contusions, and diffuse axonal injury (DAI), as these injuries are associated with high-velocity impact (**Fig. 16**). Anterior middle cranial fossa epidural hematomas, also called benign

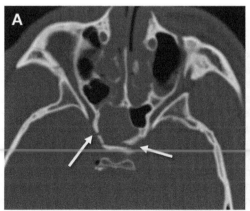

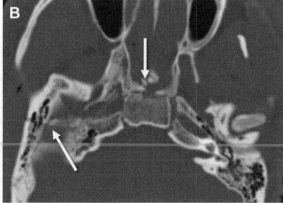

Fig. 14. Temporal bone fractures are often associated with central skull base fractures. When a temporal bone fracture is detected, careful assessment of the sphenoid sinus walls and clivus is important. Note transversely oriented fracture through the central skull base (*arrows*) extending through the sphenoid sinus walls (*A*), and extending inferiorly in the coronal plane to involve the basi sphenoid portion of the clivus and right temporal bone (*B*).

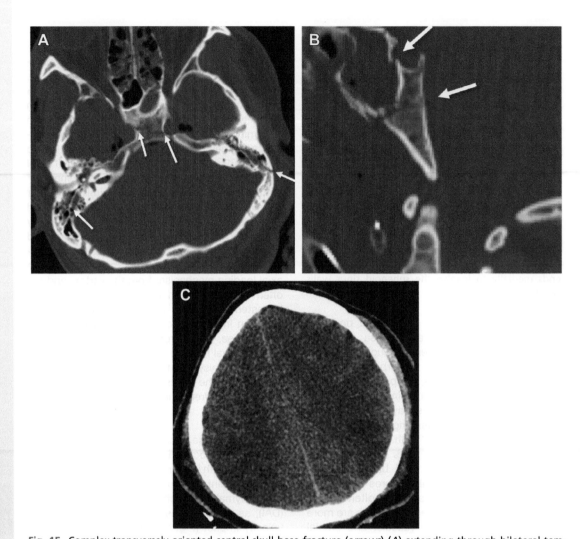

Fig. 15. Complex transversely oriented central skull base fracture (*arrows*) (*A*) extending through bilateral temporal bones, and transversely oriented through the clivus (*A, B*) and sella (*B*). The fracture extended through the carotid canals with pneumocephalus (*A*); bilateral ICA territory infarcts resulted (*C*). The patient died soon after this CT was performed.

venous epidural hematomas, occur in conjunction with injury to the greater wing of the sphenoid bone. These are postulated to be a result of venous injury to the sphenoparietal sinus, and have a benign self-limited course, not requiring surgical drainage (Fig. 17).[31] CSF leaks caused by fracture extension through the sphenoid sinus occur less frequently than in the frontobasal region, but are common with comminuted fractures.[32]

The most frequently encountered complications associated with central skull base fractures are vascular complications. Blunt cerebrovascular injury is reported in approximately 1% of all head and facial traumas, with risk increased to 8.5% in the setting of basilar skull fractures.[33–35] Fractures

extending through the central skull base are particularly at risk for ICA injury, due to this vessel's course through the central skull base and cavernous sinus. However the basilar artery is also vulnerable because of its proximity to the clivus. Overall, the fractures that are most frequently associated with vascular injury are clival fractures, fractures through the sella/sphenoid sinuses, orbital apex fractures, petrous ridge fractures, and occiput and occipital condyle fractures.[35] Fractures involving the carotid canal have an increased probability of neurovascular injury, with a positive predictive value of approximately 35% in one series (Fig. 18).[36]

The spectrum of vascular complications includes frank transection/laceration, dissection,

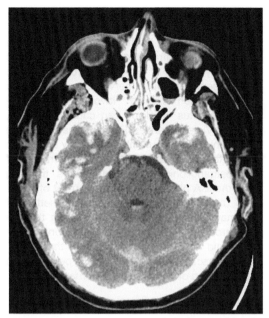

Fig. 16. Common intracranial findings associated with central skull base fractures are temporal lobe contusions, extra-axial hemorrhage, intraventricular hemorrhage, and blood within the sphenoid sinus.

vertebral artery injury. This same study showed that stroke rates decreased to 6.8% and 2.8%, respectively, for patients who received anticoagulation.[37] Therefore, early detection and treatment with anticoagulation has been the mainstay of traumatic dissection management, and screening high-risk patients with vascular imaging (most often using computed tomography angiography [CTA] or magnetic resonance angiography [MRA]) is routine.

Although cerebrovascular injury in the setting of trauma is discussed in the article by Gentry and colleagues elsewhere in this issue, the carotid cavernous fistula (CCF) deserves special mention, as it is a rare but unique complication associated with transverse or oblique central skull base fractures, occurring in 3.8% of all basilar skull fractures in one series.[38] CCF presents as a traumatic direct connection between the ICA and the cavernous sinus, forming a high-flow fistula. Clinical presentation is with exophthalmos, bruit, chemosis, vision loss, and ophthalmoplegia, with potential resulting blindness, stroke, or death. Symptoms of CCF may present acutely, within hours of the injury, or in a delayed fashion, weeks to months after the injury. Clinical detection may be difficult in comatose or intubated patients, and a high index of suspicion should be present in patients with middle cranial fossa fractures. CCFs are treated most frequently with endovascular therapies using detachable balloon coil or other embolic materials, or with covered stent placement in an attempt to preserve ICA flow.[39]

aneurysm/pseudoaneurysm, incarceration (entrapment in a fracture line) or dural arteriovenous (AV) fistula (most commonly carotid cavernous fistula). Stroke from thromboembolic disease due to arterial dissection is reported in 31% in the setting of blunt carotid artery injury and 14% with blunt

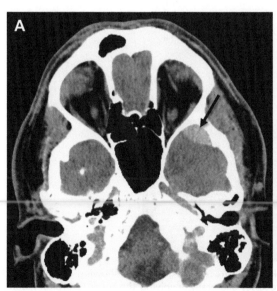

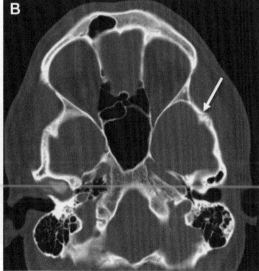

Fig. 17. (A) Epidural hematoma at anterior left middle cranial fossa (*black arrow*), adjacent to fracture line on axial CT (*arrow on B*). This most likely represents a venous epidural hematoma related to sphenoparietal sinus injury. These often have a benign, self-limited course, not requiring surgical drainage.

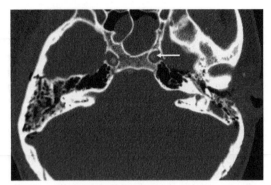

Fig. 18. Axial CTA demonstrating left temporal bone fracture extending through the left carotid canal. Note left ICA irregularity and narrowing (*arrow*), consistent with dissection.

Cranial nerve deficits may present in an acute fashion, often due to cranial nerve laceration, or in a delayed fashion, possibly because of neuronal stretching or edema. More delayed presentation injuries are associated with a better prognosis for recovery of symptoms. Fractures extending through the clinoid process and the superior orbital fissure may present with a syndrome of third, fourth, and sixth nerve palsies, as well as anesthesia in V1 distribution. Decreasing visual acuity owing to compression of the optic nerve is the hallmark of the orbital apex syndrome. Both of these clinical syndromes may necessitate

surgical decompression to preserve cranial nerve function, particularly if the fractures are comminuted and impinging on the optic nerve, or if there is a hematoma contributing to a compressive optic neuropathy (**Fig. 19**).[40] Fractures through the sella may present with optic nerve compression and bitemporal hemianopsia. Involvement of the cavernous sinus or clivus can cause CN III, IV, V1, V2, or VI neuropathies. Partial Horner syndrome (ptosis, miosis, without anhidrosis) may develop in the posttraumatic setting because of interruption of the postganglionic sympathetic fibers traveling along the ICA plexus. Although this most often reflects dissection in the posttraumatic setting, it also may result from fracture extending through the petrous portion of the temporal bone, along the carotid canal, or in the region of the Meckel cave.[41] Vascular imaging should be performed in the evaluation of posttraumatic Horner syndrome.

Posterior Skull Base Fractures

Classification/Etiology
Most posterior cranial fossa fractures occur as a result of a lateral and/or posterior blow to the occiput, and involve the occipital bone with frequent extension to the petrous temporal bone. No simple classification scheme exists for the description of all posterior skull base fractures.

Temporal bone fractures are often treated independently, and described as either transverse

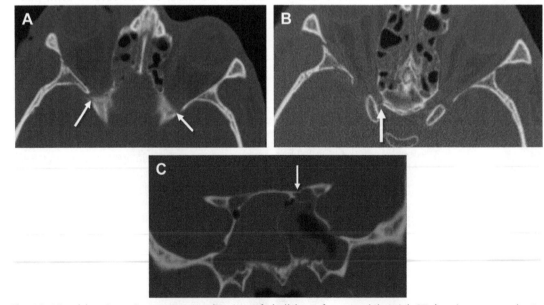

Fig. 19. Visual loss is an important complication of skull base fracture. (*A*) Axial CT showing a comminuted fracture extending through the base of the clinoid processes bilaterally, involving the superior orbital fissures (*arrows*). (*B*) Axial CT of another patient demonstrating fracture line traversing the right optic nerve canal (*arrow*). (*C*) Coronal CT of another patient demonstrating fracture extending through the left optic nerve canal (*arrow*).

or longitudinal, or otic capsule sparing or violating.[42,43] These are described in the article by Kennedy and colleagues elsewhere in this issue. Fractures involving the clivus (basi occiput) inferiorly have been discussed previously. Occipital condyle fractures are rare, and are classified by the imaging appearance and presumed mechanism as either type 1 (impacted condyle with comminution, due to axial loading), type 2 (basilar skull fracture with linear extension into the occipital condyle), or type 3 (avulsion fracture at the attachment site for the alar ligaments) (**Fig. 20**).[44]

Complications

Posterior skull base fractures are frequently associated with posterior fossa intracranial injuries, including extradural, subdural, and cerebellar parenchymal hematomas. Posterior fossa epidural hematomas are the most frequently encountered complication associated with posterior skull base fractures, and are often venous due to injury to the transverse or sigmoid dural venous sinuses or the jugular bulb. These are more frequently seen in children and can expand rapidly, leading to sudden clinical deterioration from fourth ventricular or brainstem compression. Early diagnosis and management is imperative (**Fig. 21**). Small hematomas without mass effect may be managed conservatively with clinical and radiologic follow-up, whereas larger hematomas with mass effect often require decompression.[45–47]

Posterior skull base fractures through the venous sinuses or jugular foramen causing venous sinus injury can also predispose to venous sinus thrombosis or the long-term complication of dural AV fistula. Venous sinus thrombosis can present with worsening intracranial hypertension, venous infarctions, or hemorrhage.[48] Follow-up studies demonstrating increased density in the expected location of the venous sinuses should prompt evaluation with CT venography (**Fig. 22**).

Lower cranial nerve injuries may occur in posterior skull base fractures, again depending on the location and pattern of injury. Temporal bone fractures may be associated with both CN VII and VIII injuries. Facial paralysis, along with CSF leak, is one of the most common indications for surgical intervention in temporal bone fractures. Transverse fractures through the temporal bone are more commonly associated with facial paresis than longitudinal fractures, with injury typically at the level of the internal auditory canal or labyrinthine segments. When facial nerve injury occurs in the setting of longitudinal fractures, it is most commonly at the level of the geniculate ganglion (**Fig. 23**).[40,42,43] Fractures extending through the jugular foramen, in addition to causing vascular injury or thrombosis, also predispose to glossopharyngeal, vagal, or spinal accessory nerve injuries, resulting in dysphagia with loss of the gag reflex, ipsilateral vocal cord paralysis with hoarseness, and paralysis of the ipsilateral sternocleidomastoid and trapezius musculature (**Fig. 24**). Fracture through the hypoglossal canal, as can be seen with adjacent occipital condyle injuries, can predispose to ipsilateral tongue deviation and hemiatrophy (**Fig. 25**).[40,49,50]

As with anterior cranial fossa fractures, comminuted fractures through the temporal bones may be complicated by CSF leaks with or without associated meningoencephaloceles, particularly if the fractures are displaced through the tegmen tympani or mastoideum, or along the posterior petrous ridge. These fractures may result in CSF

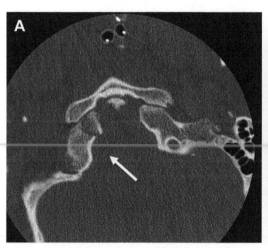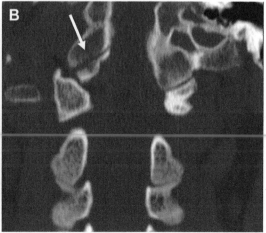

Fig. 20. Axial (*A*) and Coronal (*B*) CT images demonstrating a mildly diastatic type III avulsion fracture of the right occipital condyle (*arrows*).

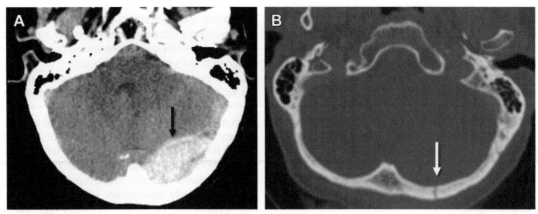

Fig. 21. (*A*) Axial soft tissue window through the posterior fossa demonstrating a large epidural hematoma (*black arrow*), causing mass effect on the fourth ventricle. (*B*) Bone window CT image shows the underlying occipital bone fracture (*arrow*).

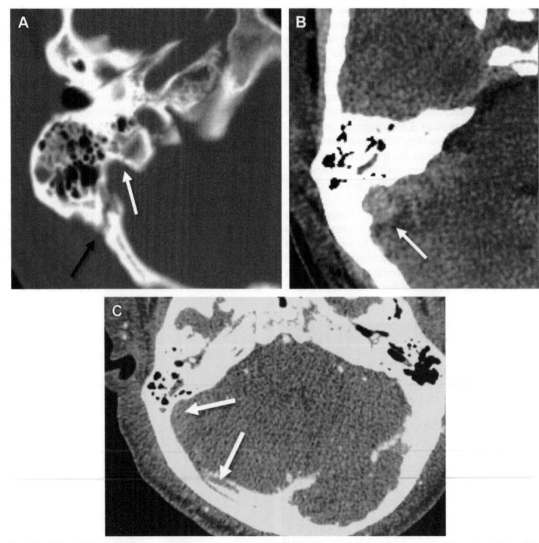

Fig. 22. (*A*) Axial CT image through the right temporal bone and posterior fossa showing diastasis of the right occipitomastoid suture (*black arrow*), with subtle fracture extending medially through the sigmoid sinus (*arrow*). (*B*) Noncontrast head CT shows increased density in the expected location of the sigmoid sinus (*arrow*). (*C*) CTA/CTV image demonstrates a clot in the right transverse and sigmoid sinus (*arrows*).

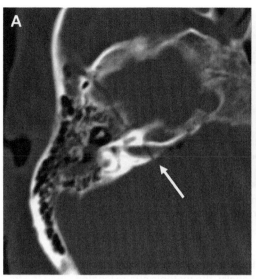
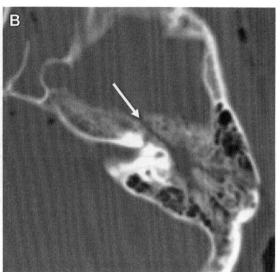

Fig. 23. Facial nerve palsy and hearing loss are complications of skull base fractures. (*A*) Medial transverse fracture (with respect to the petrous ridge) through the right temporal bone, extending through the internal auditory canal (*arrow*). (*B*) Longitudinal fracture through the left temporal bone extending through the expected location of the geniculate ganglion (*arrow*).

otorrhea or rhinorrhea (via extension through the Eustachian tube), as well as traumatic meningocele, and predispose the patient to meningitis (**Fig. 26**). As in anterior skull base trauma, presentation may be acute or delayed.

Finally, basi occiput clival and occipital condylar fractures extending through the craniocervical junction often present with vertebrobasilar injury as well as cervical spine injuries, with varying degrees of ligamentous injury and possibility for craniocervical dissociation (**Fig. 27**). Therefore, fractures in this region should prompt vascular imaging with CTA or MRA, as well as magnetic resonance imaging (MRI) of the cervical spine to assess for ligamentous injuries.[3,29,35]

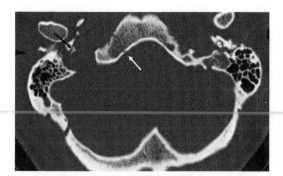

Fig. 24. Complex right posterior skull base fracture extending through the right occipital bone, along the right jugular foramen (pars vascularis) and carotid canal (*black arrow*). There is also a longitudinal fracture of the basi occiput of the clivus (*arrow*).

DIAGNOSTIC CRITERIA

In addition to more general indicators of craniofacial injury, such as low Glasgow coma scale scores, clinical findings associated with skull base fracture include periorbital ecchymosis, Battle sign (postauricular ecchymosis), hemotympanum, and CSF otorrhea or rhinorrhea.[51,52] Acute cranial nerve deficits in the setting of head trauma should raise the suspicion for skull base fracture.[53] The imaging diagnosis is made by detecting the fracture line on CT as a noncorticated, noninterdigitating lucency in skull base bone, with or without adjacent pneumocephalus, sinus or middle ear/mastoid opacification, or intraorbital emphysema.

CSF leak is most often diagnosed clinically by CSF rhinorrhea or otorrhea, clear drainage that increases with Valsalva or positional maneuvers. The gold standard confirmatory test for the presence of CSF in the rhinorrhea or otorrhea is the beta 2 transferrin assay, or the newer beta trace protein assay. These proteins are specific to CSF, and the assays confer a very high sensitivity and specificity for CSF leak, with rare false positives in the setting of liver failure. Only a few drops are required to make the diagnosis.[54,55]

DIFFERENTIAL DIAGNOSIS

Skull base fractures can often be difficult to detect on CT, particularly if linear and noncomminuted, and a thorough knowledge of skull base anatomy is necessary to avoid diagnosing

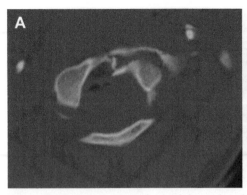

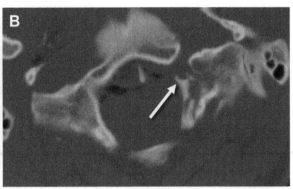

Fig. 25. This patient is at risk for both hypoglossal nerve injury and vertebral artery dissection. (*A*) Comminuted fracture of the left occipital condyle. (*B*) Note fracture fragment (*arrow*) extending into the left hypoglossal canal.

"pseudofractures." Many small neural and vascular channels and foramina that can be seen on multidetector CT (MDCT) can mimic fracture lines, as can sutures and skull base fissures. Additionally, suture lines also can become diastatic and widened after skull base injury.

In the anterior skull base, the anterior and posterior ethmoid artery canals may be confused with skull base fractures, and one should note the corticated margins and tapering nature (see **Fig. 2**B). The supraorbital canal is a characteristic notch along the medial third of the supraorbital rim, which transmits the supraorbital artery and nerve. The sphenofrontal suture as it courses along the superolateral orbit can mimic a fracture line, and one should note the interdigitating and corticated

lucency and characteristic location (**Fig. 28**). Additionally, the metopic suture located along the frontal bone in the midline can persist in up to 10% of adults as a lucency between the frontal sinuses along the interfrontal sinus septum.[56]

Within the central skull base, the vidian canal, as well as minor neurovascular channels associated with the foramen rotundum and foramen ovale, can simulate fractures. Specifically, the palatovaginal canal, a canal inferomedial to the vidian canal extending from the pterygopalatine fossa to the roof of the pharynx that carries the pterygovaginal artery (branch of the maxillary artery) and the pharyngeal nerve, can simulate a fracture on axial images (**Fig. 29**). Several canals and channels can persist within the clivus and mimic fractures.

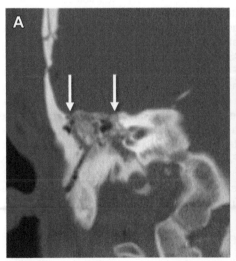

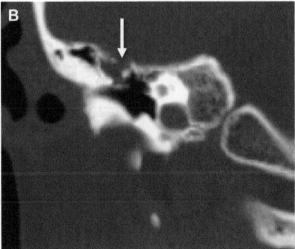

Fig. 26. Acute and chronic tegmen defects, with risk of CSF leak. (*A*) Coronal CT shows displaced and comminuted right temporal bone fractures (*arrows*) extending through the tegmen with scattered pneumocephalus. (*B*) Coronal CT of a patient with a history of remote trauma demonstrates a defect along the tegmen (*arrow*), and adjacent meningoencephalocele.

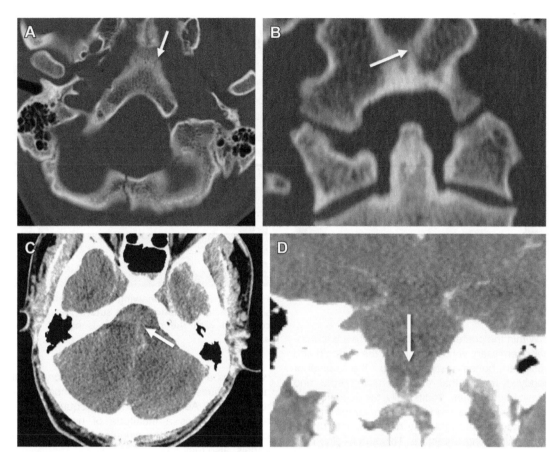

Fig. 27. CTA should be considered to assess for vascular injury in the setting of clivus fractures. Axial CT through the posterior fossa (A) showing a right paramedian occipital bone fracture extending through the foramen magnum, with a linear nondisplaced fracture extending along the left paramedian basi occiput portion of the clivus (*arrow*), in a longitudinal orientation (A, B). In spite of the relatively nondisplaced appearance of the longitudinal clivus fracture, there were devastating complications with brainstem hemorrhage (*arrow*) (C), as well as basilar artery occlusion (*arrow*) (D). The patient did not survive the injury.

Within the superior basi sphenoid clivus, the craniopharyngeal or persistent hypophyseal canal can be rarely seen in the adult as a linear longitudinally oriented canal coursing anteriorly and inferiorly from the sella toward the nasopharynx. More inferiorly within the midline of the basi occiput of the clivus, an anatomic variant, the medial basal canal (or canalis basilaris medianus) may exist, likely a notochordal remnant. The spheno-occipital synchondrosis, or transverse clival cleft, separates the basi sphenoid from the basi occiput and usually closes in teenage years, but can persist into the 20s, mimicking a transverse clival fracture. Finally, other sutures and fissures that can mimic fracture lines include the petro occipital fissure, which transmits the inferior petrosal sinus, as well as the sphenosquamosal suture (lateral to the foramen spinosum) and the sphenopetrosal synchondrosis (between the foramen ovale and the carotid canal) (**Fig. 30**).[56]

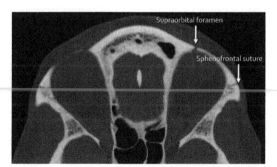

Fig. 28. Anterior cranial fossa pseudofractures, including the supraorbital foramen and the interdigitating sphenofrontal suture line characteristically located along the superolateral orbital rim.

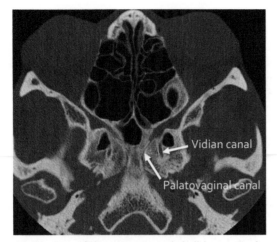

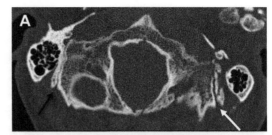

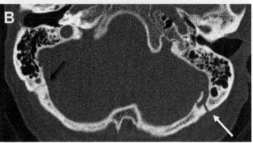

Fig. 29. One of the many central skull base pseudo-fractures, the palatovaginal canal, an inferior sphenoid bone canal extending to the pterygopalatine fossa and located inferomedial to the well-corticated vidian canal.

Fig. 31. (A, B) Axial CT showing posttraumatic diastasis of the left occipitomastoid suture line (arrow), compared with the right, which is normal (black arrow).

Within the posterior skull base, there are a number of emissary venous canals in the mastoid and occipital bones extending to the posterior condylar region that may be asymmetric and mimic fracture lines. Additionally, the occipitomastoid suture, as it extends to the jugular foramen, is often asymmetric and may have few interdigitations, mimicking a fracture. This suture also may become diastatic and widened in the setting of posterior skull base fracture (Fig. 31). There are many temporal bone pseudofractures, discussed in detail in the article by Kennedy and colleagues on temporal bone trauma elsewhere in this issue. These include the tympanomastoid suture posteriorly, as well as the tympanosquamous suture,

which lies anterior to the external auditory canal and continues medially as the petrotympanic suture (Fig. 32). Additionally, the petrosquamous suture, as well as a multitude of neurovascular channels, including the singular and subarcuate canals, also may mimic fractures.[56,57]

IMAGING FINDINGS

The first imaging modality necessary in the patient with suspected skull base trauma is a noncontrast head CT, as patients will be initially managed and triaged based on intracranial injuries. Pneumocephalus should raise suspicion for a fracture through the anterior skull base or the temporal bone. Additionally, significant or serially increasing pneumocephalus suggests a dural tear and possible CSF leak, although pneumocephalus has been reported in some cases of cranial extension of extensive subcutaneous emphysema in the absence of skull base fracture.[58]

Face CT, with multidetector thin-slice CT images through the face and skull base, also should be obtained in any patient with a suspected skull base fracture. Soft tissue windows are assessed for intraorbital emphysema, extraocular muscle injury, retrobulbar or subperiosteal hemorrhage, globe rupture, intraocular hemorrhage or lens dislocation, as well as for facial soft tissue injuries and paranasal sinus hemorrhage.

Thin-section bone algorithm images should be scrutinized and reconstructed in the coronal and sagittal planes, as multiplanar reconstruction has

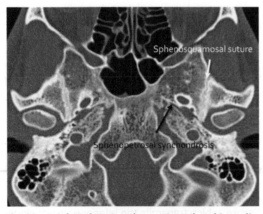

Fig. 30. Axial CT showing the corticated and interdigitating sphenosquamosal suture (arrow) lateral to the foramen spinosum, and the sphenopetrosal synchondrosis between foramen ovale and the carotid canal.

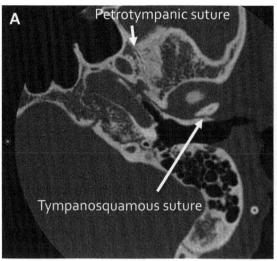
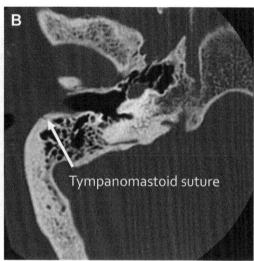

Fig. 32. Temporal bone CT images showing pseudofractures, including the tympanosquamous suture that continues medially as the petrotympanic suture (*A*), and the tympanomastoid suture (*B*).

been shown to improve fracture detection.[59] Manipulating the data on a 3-dimensional (3D) workstation and optimizing the window and level settings is often helpful. Additionally, 3D volumetric reconstruction can be useful to detect the fractures, assess any facial deformity, and to aid in surgical planning for reconstruction.[60] A skull base fracture is a noncorticated, noninterdigitating lucency through the skull base, often seen with pneumocephalus or intraorbital emphysema, and opacification and air-fluid levels in adjacent sinuses or mastoids. Displacement of bone fragments should be noted, as these can be associated with dural tear. Complex facial fractures often are associated with highly comminuted anterior cranial fossa fractures (type III frontobasal fractures). Fractures along the anterior cranial fossa, particularly along the cribriform plates and ethmoid roofs, as well as along the carotid canals, may be subtle.

Fractures through the carotid canal, particularly when there is intracanalicular air, or those extending through the clivus, should prompt evaluation with CT or MRA. Studies with 16-slice multidetector CTA have shown up to 92% negative predictive value, suggesting that CTA can replace the gold standard digital subtraction angiography (DSA) for screening of suspected blunt carotid and vertebral artery injuries.[61] Additionally, significantly enlarged superior ophthalmic veins, or asymmetric fullness or air within the cavernous sinus, should prompt vascular evaluation with CTA or DSA to assess for carotid-cavernous fistula. Any suspicion of thromboembolic disease, such as clinical or imaging findings of stroke, should prompt vascular imaging. Finally, increased density in the

expected location of venous sinuses may represent extra-axial hemorrhage or even venous sinus thrombosis, and should prompt evaluation with CT venography (CTV).

One of the most obvious imaging findings of blunt carotid and vertebral artery injury on CTA or CTV is vascular occlusion (due to occluding dissection or thromboembolic disease) with lack of vessel opacification. However, dissection or pseudoaneurysm also can be more subtle, manifesting as vessel wall irregularity, luminal narrowing, or focal tapering of the affected vessel (**Fig. 33**).[62] CCF findings include prominent early filling and enlargement of the affected cavernous sinus, with ipsilateral prominent superior ophthalmic veins, as well as proptosis and intraorbital fat stranding. Engorged inferior petrosal sinus and other draining veins also may be seen. DSA shows fistulous communication between the

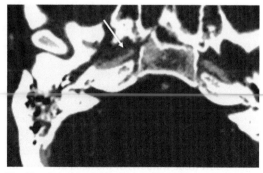

Fig. 33. CTA demonstrating right temporal bone fracture causing luminal irregularity and narrowing of the horizontal petrous segment of the right internal carotid artery (*arrow*), compatible with dissection.

carotid artery and the cavernous sinus (Fig. 34).[38] Traumatic true aneurysms, involving all of the layers of the arterial wall, also may be seen as focal outpouchings of the affected vessel, most often involving the extradural cavernous segments of the internal carotid artery in the setting of skull base fractures. Rupture of such a cavernous aneurysm may similarly result in carotid cavernous fistula formation. Other potential sites of true aneurysms include the distal cortical vessels, including the distal anterior cerebral artery pericallosal branches due to shear along the falx (Fig. 35).[63,64] Although CTA remains an adequate screening tool for vascular injury, DSA remains the gold standard for further evaluation of any suspected injuries on CTA.

MRI findings in the setting of trauma include hemorrhage and parenchymal contusion on T1-weighted, T2-weighted, gradient echo (GRE) and fluid-attenuated inversion recovery (FLAIR) images. Diffusion-weighted and GRE images can be helpful in the detection of infarction and punctate shear injury (DAI). Loss of flow voids in the vascular structures, or crescentic increased T1 and T2 signal around the periphery of the carotid or vertebral arteries, may herald vascular occlusion or dissection, respectively. Time of flight and contrast-enhanced MRA imaging findings of carotid occlusion or dissection, as well as CCF, are similar to those with CTA. The technique of dynamic contrast-enhanced MRA may be helpful in the noninvasive workup of possible CCF,

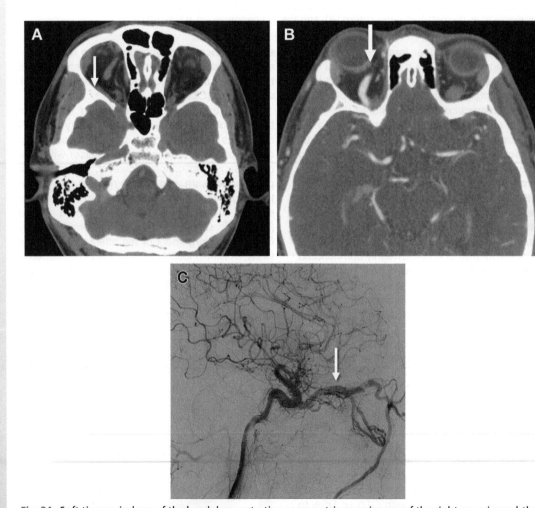

Fig. 34. Soft tissue windows of the head demonstrating asymmetric prominence of the right superior ophthalmic vein (*arrow*) (*A*), with CTA images (*B*) demonstrating early arterial enhancement of the dilated right superior ophthalmic vein (*arrow*) and mild proptosis. The findings are suggestive of carotid cavernous fistula. (*C*) Digital subtraction angiography from a right ICA injection demonstrating early filling of the cavernous sinus and enlarged superior (*arrow*) and inferior ophthalmic veins, confirming a carotid cavernous fistula.

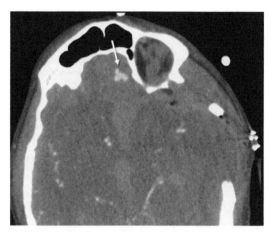

Fig. 35. Images from axial CTA demonstrating a lobulated posttraumatic aneurysm arising from the left anterior cerebral artery (*arrow*), discovered when the patient developed increased parenchymal and subarachnoid hemorrhage after a decompressive craniectomy. This complication was thought to be due to release of the initial tamponade on the ruptured aneurysm.

demonstrating early filling of the cavernous sinus and venous structures.

The imaging workup of patients presenting with symptoms of delayed CSF leak in the setting of prior trauma, including CSF rhinorrhea, otorrhea, or meningitis, should begin with thin-section high-resolution MDCT through the face and skull base, including the mastoids. Localizing the leak and characterizing the size of the skull base defect is imperative, as many repairs are performed endoscopically. MDCT has a reported 92% sensitivity for the detection of the site of the osseous defect, and is often used for intraoperative guidance for the repair.[65,66] Imaging findings suspicious for the site of CSF leak include an osseous defect or irregularity, with fluid level or opacification in the adjacent sinus. Polypoid nondependent soft tissue adjacent to the defect is characteristic of a meningoencephalocele, best assessed on MRI.[65,67] If the patient has a verified (ie, positive beta 2 transferrin) and persistent leak, and only one osseous defect and potential site of CSF leak, the imaging workup is complete, and the patient should proceed to surgery for repair.[65]

However, patients with multiple osseous defects or potential sites of CSF leak, including prior fractures through both the tegmen and the anterior skull base, may require further imaging with cisternography to determine the source of the active leak. CT cisternography with intrathecal iodinated contrast can be helpful in detecting the source of the leak; however, it requires the patient to be actively leaking, or able to elicit the leak at the time of the examination. The technique initially requires performing precontrast thin-section MDCT imaging of the sinuses and mastoids, to assess for baseline increased density in the sinus due to blood, inspissated secretions, or neo-osteogenesis. The patient then undergoes lumbar puncture with intrathecal myelographic iodinated contrast followed by repeat CT of the sinuses and mastoids after head down and provocative maneuvers in an attempt to opacify the basilar cisterns and elicit the leak. Postcontrast imaging is often performed in both prone direct coronal imaging (in an effort to elicit the leak) and supine axial acquisitions with thin-section reformations, to mimic the precontrast series. Imaging findings suggesting the site of the leak include increased density and pooling of contrast in the sinuses or mastoids adjacent to the site of an osseous defect, which also can be detected by increase in Hounsfield units on region of interest measurements. Limitations of this technique include radiation to the patient, the time-intensive nature of the interpretation comparing the precontrast and postcontrast images, the invasive nature of the procedure, with small but inherent risks related to intrathecal contrast and lumbar puncture, and that the patient must be actively leaking at the time of the study.[65]

MRI cisternography is a noninvasive, nonionizing technique using heavily T2-weighted sequences, fat-saturated spin-echo sequences, and/or high-resolution 3D T2-weighted GRE sequences through the skull base, in addition to thin-section T1 precontrast and postcontrast images in multiple planes. This technique is useful in characterizing the contents of suspected meningoencephaloceles, and can detect a CSF leak as a continuous column of T2 hyperintense material extending from the subarachnoid space into the extracranial soft tissues. Although reportedly accurate in up to 89% of cases, it is best when combined with high-resolution CT, which will still be necessary for bony detail and preoperative planning (Fig. 36).[68–70]

PITFALLS IN DETECTION OF SKULL BASE TRAUMA AND COMPLICATIONS

In addition to the overcalling of pseudofractures due to normal sutures, one of the greatest pitfalls in the imaging of skull base trauma is the failure of fracture detection. It is imperative to use multiplanar reformations, often with additional 3D reformations, in the evaluation of suspected skull base fractures, particularly in the presence of opacified sinuses or mastoids and pneumocephalus. The use of multiplanar reformations has been proven to increase fracture detection rates.[59] However, interestingly and anecdotally, there are occasions in which fracture lines and trajectories may be

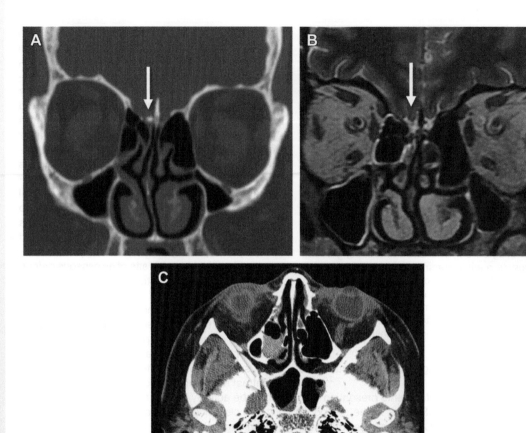

Fig. 36. (*A*) Coronal CT in a patient with a remote history of trauma and CSF rhinorrhea, with positive beta 2 transferrin, showing a defect with sclerosis along the right cribriform plate and lateral lamella (*arrow*). Another defect in the left sphenoid sinus with adjacent soft tissue was also noted, therefore the patient underwent MRI, and ultimately CT cisternography. (*B*) Coronal T2-weighted MRI image demonstrates slight sagging of the right gyrus rectus and olfactory bulb, suspicious for the site of the leak (*arrow*). Postcontrast CT cisternogram image (*C*) demonstrating pooling contrast (*arrow*) in the right posterior ethmoid, compatible with the site of the leak.

better seen on thicker-section bone algorithm images; therefore, using a combination of all of the data from thick and thin bone images is important (**Fig. 37**). One recent study recommended using curved maximum intensity projection reformations through the skull base to enhance detection rates of subtle skull base fractures.[71] Frequently missed fractures include occipital condylar fractures, subtle anterior cranial fossa fractures, and occult temporal bone fractures. Streak artifact, either from metal artifact (particularly in gunshot wound injuries) or dental amalgam can also limit evaluation of the skull base. Additionally, streak artifact through the petrous and cavernous segments of the internal carotid arteries can make evaluation on CTA challenging. Optimizing window and level settings and the use of dual-energy CT may be helpful in this setting.[72]

One of the greatest pitfalls in the imaging workup of posttraumatic CSF leaks, particularly in the delayed presentation, are those patients presenting with intermittent or suspected leaks who are unable to collect fluid for beta 2 transferrin analysis. In these patients, it is important for imaging to help confirm the diagnosis of CSF leak, as well as identify the site of the leak, particularly if high-resolution CT shows multiple osseous defects. Prior imaging modalities have been limited in the workup of these patients; however, the new technique of MRI cisternography with the administration of intrathecal gadolinium has evolved, with reported sensitivity of up to 100% for high-flow CSF leaks and 70% for intermittent leaks. In addition to the absence of ionizing radiation and relatively easy interpretation, this technique shows particular promise in the complicated

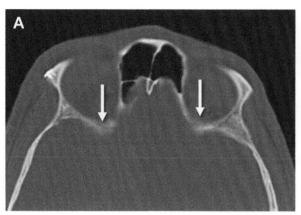
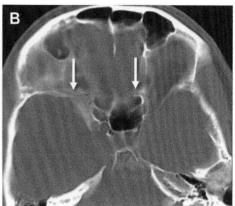

Fig. 37. Pitfall of skull base trauma imaging. Fractures may be more obvious on thicker images, but both thin and thick should be assessed. (A) A lucency is noted on the 0.625 slice thickness image (*arrows*), possibly a fracture. (B) Fracture is much better seen on the thicker 5-mm bone window image (*arrows*).

patients with intermittent leaks, due to the possibility of delayed imaging up to 24 hours after injection (**Fig. 38**).[73] However, large prospective trials and long-term safety studies are still lacking for this technique, and although most studies performed in the European literature have shown no adverse or unexpected effects with doses used, the intrathecal administration of gadolinium contrast is not currently approved by the Food and Drug Administration in the United States. Literature-based recommended algorithm for the imaging workup of chronic post-traumatic CSF leaks is described in **Fig. 39**.

WHAT THE REFERRING PHYSICIAN NEEDS TO KNOW

Regardless of classification systems used, delineating fracture extent; degree of comminution; fracture fragments; associated intracranial and intraorbital injury; and involvement of certain anatomic regions, foramina, and vascular channels is important. **Box 1** has a checklist of structures to assess in the evaluation of each skull base fracture.

In our practice, CTA/V is routinely recommended for any complex skull base fracture that involves the carotid canal, cavernous sinus, or major venous channel, including the transverse sinus, superior sagittal sinus, and jugular foramen. This imaging is done urgently, as soon as the fracture is detected, often before the patient leaves the emergency room and is admitted to the surgical intensive care unit. We are careful to coordinate the imaging and intravenous contrast doses, as patients with multiple trauma often undergo contrast CT of the abdomen and chest as well as the brain. If an arterial injury is present, the vascular neurologist is consulted, as anticoagulation in the trauma

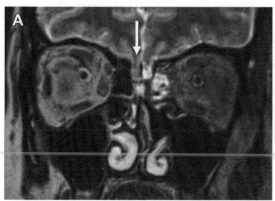
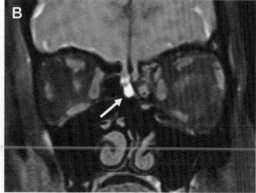

Fig. 38. Patient with intermittent CSF leak, and history of prior trauma. (A) Coronal T2-weighted images from noncontrast MRI cisternography demonstrating sagging of the right gyrus rectus (*arrow*), with adjacent T2 hyperintensity in the superior nasal cavity, suspicious for a meningocele. A second defect (not shown) was also present and MRI cisternography was requested to determine the source of the leak. (B) Fat-saturated T1-weighted image from MRI cisternogram after intrathecal gadolinium demonstrates contrast opacification of the small right meningocele (*arrow*). The left ethmoid sinuses do not fill with contrast, so the secretions are not CSF.

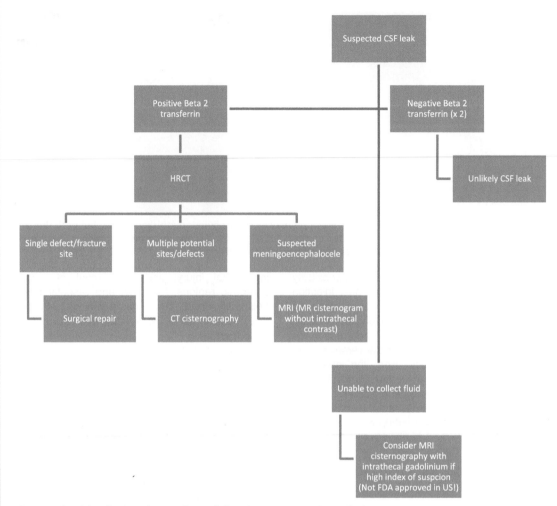

Fig. 39. Algorithm for imaging workup of chronic posttraumatic CSF leak.

Box 1
What the referring physicians need to know

Checklist of sites to assess for skull base fracture involvement.

  Posterior table of frontal sinus

  Anterior skull base

  Optic canal

  Superior orbital fissure

  Skull base foramina involvement (ie, foramen rotundum/ovale)

  Carotid canal

  Sigmoid sinus/jugular foramen

  Tegmen

  Clivus

  Occipital condyle

  Hypoglossal canal

---

patient is possible, despite intracranial and abdominal hematomas, but the risk versus benefit must be considered.

CSF leak, on the other hand, is a complication that is considered later, in the rehabilitation period. Most small dural defects close spontaneously and require no advanced imaging. Cranial nerve injury, especially the facial nerve, should be diagnosed in the acute to subacute period, using a combination of the clinical examination and imaging, so that neural repair can be considered.

FUTURE CONSIDERATIONS/SUMMARY

Skull base fractures are a frequent complication of high-impact trauma, and due to the inherent anatomic relationships of the skull base, even relatively linear nondisplaced fractures may be associated with significant intracranial complications, including CSF leak; therefore, their detection is important. Additionally, continued improvement in endoscopic techniques have led to fewer open surgeries for repair, necessitating better and more accurate assessment of skull base fractures and resultant defects. MDCT scanner and reconstruction software improvements will likely continue to facilitate fracture detection, with the faster, newer-generation scanners allowing for less motion, and contributing to better CTA techniques. Dual-energy CT may be helpful in the future as well. Finally, MRI with intrathecal gadolinium is a promising new technique for the evaluation of CSF leak, particularly in the setting of intermittent or suspected leaks.

REFERENCES

1. National Trauma Data Bank. Annual report, 2013. Available at: http://www.facs.org/trauma/ntdb/pdf/ntdb-annual-report-2013.pdf. Accessed November, 2013.

2. Yilmazlar S, Arslan E, Kocaeli H, et al. Cerebrospinal fluid leakage complicating skull base fractures: analysis of 81 cases. Neurosurg Rev 2006;29:64–71.

3. Samii M, Tatgiba M. Skull base trauma: diagnosis and management. Neurol Res 2002;24:147–56.

4. Manson PN, Stanwix MG, Yaremchuk MJ, et al. Frontobasal fractures: anatomical classification and clinical significance. Plast Reconstr Surg 2009;124:2096–106.

5. Madhusudan G, Sharma RK, Kanhdelwal N, et al. Nomenclature of frontobasal trauma: a new clinicoradiographic classification. Plast Reconstr Surg 2006;117:2382–8.

6. Piccirilli M, Anichini G, Cassoni A, et al. Anterior cranial fossa traumas: clinical value, surgical indications, and results—a retrospective study on a series of 223 patients. J Neurol Surg B Skull Base 2012;73:265–72.

7. Bell RB, Chen J. Frontobasilar fractures: contemporary management. Atlas Oral Maxillofac Surg Clin North Am 2010;18(2):181–96.

8. Guy WM, Brissett AE. Contemporary management of traumatic fracture of the frontal sinus. Otolaryngol Clin North Am 2013;46:733–48.

9. Chaaban MR, Conger B, Riley KO, et al. Transnasal endoscopic repair of posterior table fractures. Otolaryngol Head Neck Surg 2012;147(6):1142–7.

10. Pease M, Marquez Y, Tuchman A, et al. Diagnosis and surgical management of traumatic cerebrospinal fluid oculorrhea: case report and systematic review of the literature. J Neurol Surg Rep 2013;74: 57–66.

11. Aarabi B, Leibrock LG. Neurosurgical approaches to cerebrospinal fluid rhinorrhea. Ear Nose Throat J 1992;71(7):300–5.

12. Ziu M, Savage JG, Jimenez DG. Diagnosis and treatment of cerebrospinal fluid rhinorrhea following accidental traumatic anterior skull base fractures. Neurosurg Focus 2012;32(6):1–17.

13. Eljamel MS, Foy PM. Acute traumatic CSF fistulae: the risk of intracranial infection. Br J Neurosurg 1990;4(5):381–5.

14. Ratilal B, Costa J, Sampaio C, et al. Antibiotic prophylaxis for preventing meningitis in patients with basilar skull fractures. Cochrane Database Syst Rev 2011;(8):CD004884.

15. Wax MK, Ramadan HH, Ortiz O, et al. Contemporary management of cerebrospinal fluid rhinorrhea. Otolaryngol Head Neck Surg 1997;116:442–9.

16. Schlosser RJ, Bolger WE. Nasal cerebrospinal fluid leaks: critical review and surgical considerations. Laryngoscope 2004;114:255–65.

17. Mincy JE. Posttraumatic cerebrospinal fluid fistulae of the frontal fossa. J Trauma 1966;6:618–22.

18. Bell RB, Dierks EJ, Homer L, et al. Management of cerebrospinal fluid leak associated with craniomaxillofacial trauma. J Oral Maxillofac Surg 2004;62(6): 676–84.

19. Savva A, Taylor MJ, Beatty CW. Management of cerebrospinal fluid leak involving the temporal bone: report on 92 patients. Laryngoscope 2003;113: 50–6.

20. Abrishamkar S, Khalighinejad N, Moein P. Analysing the effect of early acetazolaminde administration on patients with a high risk of permanent cerebrospinal fluid leakage. Acta Med Iran 2013; 51(7):467–71.

21. Rocchi G, Caroli E, Belli E, et al. Severe craniofacial fractures with frontobasal involvement and cerebrospinal fluid fistula: indications for surgical repair. Surg Neurol 2005;63:559–64.

22. Scholsem M, Scholtes F, Collignon F, et al. Surgical management of anterior cranial base fractures with cerebrospinal fluid fistulae: a single institution experience. Neurosurgery 2008;62:463–71.

23. Villalobos T, Arango C, Kubilis P, et al. Antibiotic prophylaxis after basilar skull fractures: a meta-analysis. Clin Infect Dis 1998;27:364–9.

24. Jimenez DF, Sundrani S, Barone CM. Posttraumatic anosmia in craniofacial trauma. J Craniomaxillofac Trauma 1997;3(1):8–15.

25. West OC, Mirvis SE, Shanmuganathan K. Transsphenoid basilar skull fracture: CT patterns. Radiology 1993;188(2):329–38.

26. Ali QM, Dietrich B, Becker H. Patterns of skull base fracture: a three-dimensional computed tomographic study. Neuroradiology 1994;36(8):622–4.

27. Ochalski PG, Spiro RM, Fabio A, et al. Fractures of the clivus: a contemporary series in the computed tomography era. Neurosurgery 2009;65(6): 1063–9.

28. Menkü A, Koç RK, Tucer B, et al. Clivus fractures: clinical presentations and courses. Neurosurg Rev 2004;27(3):194–8.

29. Taguchi Y, Matsuzawa M, Morishima H, et al. Incarceration of the basilar artery in a longitudinal fracture of the clivus: case report and literature review. J Trauma 2000;48(6):1148–52.

30. Antoniades K, Karakasis D, Taskos N. Abducens nerve palsy following transverse fracture of the middle cranial fossa. J Craniomaxillofac Surg 1993;21(4):172–5.

31. Gean AD, Fischbein NJ, Purcell DD, et al. Benign anterior temporal epidural hematoma: indolent lesion with a characteristic CT imaging appearance after blunt head trauma. Radiology 2010; 257(1):212–8.

32. Lin DT, Lin AC. Surgical treatment of traumatic injuries of the cranial base. Otolaryngol Clin North Am 2013;46:749–57.

33. Berne JD, Cook A, Rowe SA, et al. A multivariate logistic regression analysis of risk factors for blunt cerebrovascular injury. J Vasc Surg 2010;51:57–64.

34. Mundinger GS, Dorafshar AH, Gilson MM, et al. Blunt-mechanism facial fracture patterns associated with internal carotid artery injuries: recommendations for additional screening criteria based on analysis of 4,398 patients. J Oral Maxillofac Surg 2013;71(12):2092–100.

35. Feiz-Erfan I, Horn EM, Theodore N, et al. Incidence and pattern of direct blunt neurovascular injury associated with trauma to the skull base. J Neurosurg 2007;107(2):364–9.

36. York G, Barboriak D, Petrella J, et al. Association of internal carotid artery injury with carotid canal fractures in patients with head trauma. Am J Roentgenol 2005;184(5):1672–8.

37. Miller PR, Fabian TC, Bee TK, et al. Blunt cerebrovascular injuries: diagnosis and treatment. J Trauma 2001;51:279–85.

38. Liang W, Xiaofeng Y, Weiguo L, et al. Traumatic carotid cavernous fistula accompanying basilar skull fracture: a study on the incidence of traumatic carotid cavernous fistula in the patients with basilar skull fracture and the prognostic analysis about traumatic carotid cavernous fistula. J Trauma 2007;693(5):1014–20.

39. Gemmete JJ, Ansari SA, Ghandi DM. Endovascular techniques for treatment of carotid cavernous fistula. J Neuroophthalmol 2009;29(1):62–71.

40. Katzen JT, Jarrahy R, Eby JB, et al. Craniofacial and skull base trauma. J Trauma 2003;54:1026–34.

41. Worthington JP, Snape L. Horner's syndrome secondary to a basilar skull fracture after maxillofacial trauma. J Oral Maxillofac Surg 1998;56(8):996–1000.

42. Dahiya R, Keller JD, Litofsky NS, et al. Temporal bone fractures: otic capsule sparing versus otic capsule violating clinical and radiographic considerations. J Trauma 1999;47:1079–83.

43. Johnson F, Semaan MT, Megerian CA. Temporal bone fracture: evaluation and management in the modern era. Otolaryngol Clin North Am 2008;41: 597–618.

44. Maddox JJ, Rodriguez-Feo JA, Maddox GE, et al. Nonoperative treatment of occipital condyle fractures. Spine 2012;37:E964–8.

45. Karasu A, Sabanci PA, Izgi N, et al. Traumatic epidural hematomas of the posterior cranial fossa. Surg Neurol 2008;69:247–52.

46. Blaik V, Lehto H, Hoza D, et al. Posterior fossa extradural hematomas. Cent Eur Neurosurg 2010;71: 167–72.

47. Takeuchi S, Takasato Y, Wada K, et al. Traumatic posterior fossa subdural hematomas. J Trauma 2012;72:480–6.

48. Zhao X, Rizzo A, Malek B, et al. Basilar skull fracture: a risk factor for transverse/sigmoid venous sinus obstruction. J Neurotrauma 2008;25(2):104–11.

49. Huang HH, Fang TJ, Li HY, et al. Vagus nerve paralysis due to skull base fracture. Auris Nasus Larynx 2008;35(1):153–5.

50. Lehn AC, Lettieri J, Grimley R. A case of bilateral lower cranial nerve palsies after base of skull trauma with complex management issues: case report and review of the literature. Neurologist 2012;18(3):152–4.

51. Pretto Flores L, De Almeida CS, Casulari LA. Positive predictive values of selected clinical signs associated with skull base fractures. J Neurosurg Sci 2000;44(2):77–82.

52. Somasundaram A, Laxton AW, Perrin RG. The clinical features of periorbital ecchymosis in a series of trauma patients. Injury 2014;45:203–5.

53. Krishnan DG. Systematic assessment of the patient with facial trauma. Oral Maxillofac Surg Clin North Am 2013;25:537–44.

54. Bleier BS, Debnath I, O'Connell BP. Preliminary study on the stability of beta-2 transferrin in extracorporeal CSF. Otolaryngol Head Neck Surg 2011;144:101–3.

55. Sampaio MH, de Barros-Mazon S, Sakano E, et al. Predictability of quantification of beta-trace protein for diagnosis of cerebrospinal fluid leak: cutoff determination in nasal fluids with two control groups. Am J Rhinol Allergy 2009;23(6):585–90.

56. Connor SE, Tan G, Fernando R, et al. Computed tomography pseudofractures of the mid face and skull base. Clin Radiol 2005;60:1268–79.

57. Kwong Y, Yu D, Shah J. Fracture mimics on temporal bone CT: a guide for the radiologist. AJR Am J Roentgenol 2012;199:428–34.

58. Choi YY, Hyun DK, Park HC, et al. Pneumocephalus in the absence of craniofacial skull base fracture. J Trauma 2009;66:E24–7.

59. Connor SE, Flis C. The contribution of high-resolution multiplanar reformats of the skull base to the detection of skull base fractures. Clin Radiol 2005;60:878–85.

60. Ringl H, Schernthaner R, Philipp MO, et al. Three dimensional fracture visualization of multidetector CT of the skull base in trauma patients: comparison of three reconstruction algorithms. Eur Radiol 2009; 19:2416–24.

61. Utter GH, Hollingworth W, Hallam DK, et al. Sixteen slice CT angiography in patients with suspected blunt carotid and vertebral artery injuries. J Am Coll Surg 2006;203:838–48.

62. Vertinsky AT, Schwartz NE, Fischbein NJ, et al. Comparison of multidetector CT angiography and MR imaging of cervical artery dissection. AJNR Am J Neuroradiol 2008;29:1753–60.

63. Uzan M, Cantasdemir M, Seckin MS, et al. Traumatic intracranial carotid tree aneurysms. Neurosurgery 1998;43(6):1314–20.

64. Nakstad PH, Gjertsen O, Pedersen HK. Correlation of head trauma and traumatic aneurysms. Interv Neuroradiol 2008;14:33–8.

65. Lloyd KM, Delgaudio JM, Hudgins PA. Imaging of skull base cerebrospinal fluid leaks in adults. Radiology 2008;248(3):725–36.

66. Lloyd MN, Kimber PM, Burrows EH. Post-traumatic cerebrospinal fluid rhinorrhoea: modern high-definition computed tomography is all that is required for the effective demonstration of the site of leakage. Clin Radiol 1994;49(2): 100–3.

67. Manes RP, Ryan MW, Marple BF. A novel finding on computed tomography in the diagnosis and localization of cerebrospinal fluid leaks without a clear bony defect. Int Forum Allergy Rhinol 2012;2(5): 402–4. http://dx.doi.org/10.1002/alr.21048.

68. El Gammal T, Brooks BS. MR cisternography: initial experience in 41 cases. AJNR Am J Neuroradiol 1994;15(9):1647–56.

69. Shetty PG, Shroff MM, Sahani DV, et al. Evaluation of high-resolution CT and MR cisternography in the diagnosis of cerebrospinal fluid fistula. AJNR Am J Neuroradiol 1998;19:633–9.

70. El Gammal T, Sobol W, Wadlington VR, et al. Cerebrospinal fluid fistula: detection with MR cisternography. AJNR Am J Neuroradiol 1998;19:627–31.

71. Ringl H, Schernthaner RE, Schueller G, et al. The skull unfolded: a cranial CT visualization algorithm for fast and easy detection of skull fractures. Radiology 2010;255(2):553–62.

72. Stolzmann P, Winklhofer S, Schwendener N. Monoenergetic computed tomography reconstructions reduce beam hardening artifacts from dental restorations. Forensic Sci Med Pathol 2013;9(3): 327–32.

73. Selcuk H, Albayram S, Ozer H, et al. Intrathecal gadolinium-enhanced MR cisternography in the evaluation of CSF leakage. AJNR Am J Neuroradiol 2010;31:71–5.

Imaging of Temporal Bone Trauma

Tabassum A. Kennedy, MD*, Gregory D. Avey, MD, Lindell R. Gentry, MD

KEYWORDS

- Temporal bone fracture • Trauma • Ossicular injury • Hearing loss • Facial nerve
- Cerebrospinal fluid leak • Pneumolabyrinth • Perilymphatic fistula

KEY POINTS

- Multidetector temporal bone computed tomography examinations should be performed in patients with a clinical or radiographic suspicion of temporal bone fracture.
- Categorization of temporal bone fractures should include a descriptor for fracture direction, the presence or absence of labyrinthine involvement, and the segment of temporal bone involved.
- It is important to identify associated complications related to temporal bone trauma that will guide management. Complications include injury to the tympanic membrane, ossicular chain, vestibulo-cochlear apparatus, facial nerve, tegmen, carotid canal, and venous system.

INTRODUCTION

The temporal bone is at risk for injury in the setting of high-impact craniofacial trauma occurring in 3% to 22% of patients with trauma with skull fractures (Table 1).[1–3] Motor vehicle collisions, assaults, and falls are the most common mechanisms of injury.[4–6] Most patients with temporal bone trauma sustain unilateral injury, occurring in 80% to 90% of cases.[5,7,8] Multidetector computed tomography (CT) has revolutionized the ability to evaluate the intricate anatomy of the temporal bone, enabling clinicians to detect fractures and complications related to temporal bone trauma. An understanding of temporal bone anatomy is crucial in evaluating patients with trauma for temporal bone injury; this is beyond the scope of this article, but discussed in detail by Davidson.[9]

TEMPORAL BONE IMAGING

Patients presenting to the emergency department with significant head trauma should undergo initial evaluation with a noncontrast CT examination of the head. Careful scrutiny of the temporal bone on head CT is necessary to detect primary and secondary signs of temporal bone injury. External auditory canal opacification, otomastoid opacification, air within the temporomandibular joint, ectopic intracranial air adjacent to the temporal bone, and pneumolabyrinth in the setting of trauma should raise the suspicion of an associated temporal bone fracture (Fig. 1). Patients with temporal bone trauma often sustain concomitant intracranial injury, which often necessitates more emergent management. Once life-threatening injuries are addressed, further characterization of temporal bone fracture patterns and associated complications should be performed using a checklist approach (Boxes 1 and 2). A dedicated temporal bone CT examination should be considered in those patients with clinical findings worrisome for temporal bone injury as well as those patients in whom a temporal bone fracture is suspected on imaging of the head, cervical spine, or maxillofacial region.

The authors have no financial disclosures.
Department of Radiology, Clinical Science Center, University of Wisconsin-Madison, 600 Highland Avenue, Madison, WI 53792, USA
* Corresponding author.
E-mail address: tkennedy@uwhealth.org

Neuroimag Clin N Am 24 (2014) 467–486
http://dx.doi.org/10.1016/j.nic.2014.03.003
1052-5149/14/$ – see front matter © 2014 Elsevier Inc. All rights reserved.

Table 1
Complications of temporal bone trauma based on symptoms

Symptom	Associated Imaging Finding
CHL	Tympanic membrane perforation Hemotympanum Ossicular injury (suspected in patients with persistent ABG of >30 dB for longer than 6 wk)
SNHL	Injury of the bony labyrinth Injury of the internal auditory canal Brainstem/nerve root entry zone injury Pneumolabyrinth
Vertigo	Injury of the bony labyrinth Injury of the internal auditory canal Brainstem/nerve root entry zone injury Pneumolabyrinth
Perilymphatic fistula (combination of vertigo, CHL, SNHL, possible otorrhea)	Fracture/dislocation of the stapes footplate-oval window Fracture that traverses the round window Unexplained middle ear fluid Pneumolabyrinth
Otorrhea	CSF leak related to fracture of the tegmen Violation of the stapes footplate-oval window Violation of the round window
Facial nerve weakness	Fracture, bony spicule, or hemorrhage that involves the facial nerve canal

Abbreviations: ABG, air bone gap; CHL, conductive hearing loss; CSF, cerebrospinal fluid; SNHL, sensorineural hearing loss.

The advent of multidetector CT has enabled the radiologist to critically evaluate the temporal bone in patients with trauma because of extremely fast acquisition times, very thin slices, and the ability to create multiplanar reconstructions. Axial images should be acquired using sub–1-mm slice thickness and a small field of view (<10 cm). Multiplanar reconstructions in the coronal plane, Stenvers view (oblique coronal orientation parallel to the petrous ridge), and Pöschl view (oblique coronal orientation perpendicular to the petrous ridge) can be generated for additional evaluation and cross-referencing.

FRACTURE CLASSIFICATION
Traditional Classification: Longitudinal and Transverse

In the past, temporal bone fractures were classified based on the orientation of the fracture plane with respect to the long axis of the petrous portion of the temporal bone (Figs. 2 and 3).[5,6,10] Fractures were characterized as longitudinal if parallel to the petrous pyramid and transverse if perpendicular to the petrous ridge (see Figs. 2 and 3).[6] A mixed subtype was subsequently incorporated into this scheme if there were components of both fracture planes. This classification scheme,

based on fracture direction, was devised from cadaveric studies and has been scrutinized for clinical usefulness.[1,6,8] Longitudinal fractures occur more frequently, ranging from 50% to 80%.[6–8] Transverse fractures are less common and have been reported to occur in 10% to 20% of cases.[6–8] Some clinicians think that classifying fractures as longitudinal or transverse based on axial imaging is arbitrary, because most fractures are more complex in 3 dimensions.[5] A mixed or oblique subtype has been reported to occur in approximately 10% to 75% of cases.[1,5–8] The broad range seen with the mixed and oblique fracture subtypes in part reflects differences in definitions used between studies.

Alternative Classification Schemes

Subsequent studies have shown that other classification schemes that incorporate involvement of the labyrinthine structures may offer more clinical usefulness, potentially predicting those patients at higher risk for long-term sensorineural hearing loss (SNHL), intracranial injury, vascular injury, and facial nerve paralysis.[1,4] The otic capsule (bony labyrinth) is involved in a small minority of patients, occurring in only approximately 2% to 7% of cases in patients with temporal bone fracture (see Figs. 2 and 3).[1,4,8,11] However, the associated

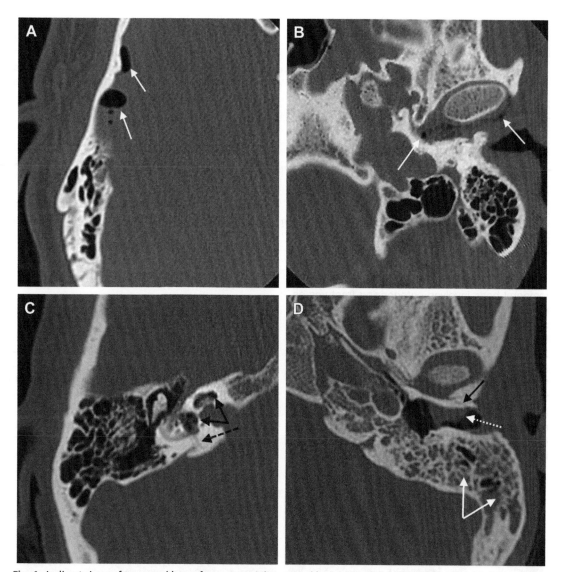

Fig. 1. Indirect signs of temporal bone fracture. Axial temporal bone CT images of 4 patients (*A–D*) show indirect signs of temporal bone fractures. Intracranial air (*A, arrows*) can be seen if the temporal bone fracture communicates with the intracranial cavity. Air within the temporomandibular joint (*B, arrows*) is often seen if the temporal bone fracture involves the tympanic ring. Pneumolabyrinth (*C, solid arrows*) can be seen if the fracture extends through the otic capsule (*C, dashed arrow*) or if there is dislocation of the stapediovestibular joint. Opacification of the mastoid air cells (*D, solid white arrows*) or external auditory canal (*D, dashed white arrow*) in the setting of trauma should raise the suspicion of an underlying temporal bone fracture involving the mastoid or tympanic ring (*D, black arrow*) respectively.

Box 1
Indirect signs of temporal bone fracture
Intracranial air adjacent to the temporal bone
Air within the temporomandibular joint
Pneumolabyrinth
Opacification of the mastoid air cells
Opacification of the external auditory canal

morbidity in patients with intralabyrinthine fractures is greater than if the otic capsule is spared.[1,8] A significant force is needed to fracture the strong bony labyrinth compared with the other weaker segments of the temporal bone. Therefore, patients with an intralabyrinthine fracture are more likely to sustain greater traumatic forces and proportionally more severe complications.

In 2004, Ishman and Friedland[8] proposed a new classification system based on the segment of

---

Box 2
Temporal bone trauma checklist

- Location and direction of temporal bone fracture
- Violation of otic capsule: cochlea, vestibule, semicircular canals, vestibular aqueduct
- Ossicular integrity: malleus, incus, stapes
- Facial nerve canal: internal auditory canal, fallopian canal, geniculate fossa, tympanic, mastoid
- Tegmen: tympani, mastoideum
- Vascular: carotid canal (petrous, cavernous), venous sinus (transverse, sigmoid, jugular bulb)

---

overall fracture pattern with additional more clinically relevant details that better anticipate associated complications. It is the identification of complications related to temporal bone trauma more than the categorization of fracture patterns that dictates how patients are managed.[12]

COMPLICATIONS

Associated complications of temporal bone trauma include injury to the tympanic membrane, ossicular chain, facial nerve, cochlea, vestibule, tegmen, and vascular structures. Patients with temporal bone trauma may present with a myriad of clinical symptoms including conductive hearing loss (CHL), SNHL, facial paralysis, CSF leak, meningitis, vertigo, and intracranial hemorrhage.

temporal bone involved categorizing fractures as petrous or nonpetrous. In this location-specific classification system, a stronger correlation between petrous-type fractures and the presence of SNHL, facial nerve injury, and cerebrospinal fluid (CSF) leak was identified. Table 2 summarizes the recent literature on temporal bone classification systems. Therefore, a combined approach incorporating a descriptor for direction (longitudinal, transverse, oblique, or mixed), temporal bone location, as well involvement of the bony labyrinth is advocated in that it provides information on the

Hearing Loss

The most common complication following temporal bone trauma is hearing loss, which is found in approximately 24% to 81% of patients with temporal bone trauma.[1,4,7,11] Hearing loss may be categorized as conductive, sensorineural, or mixed. CHL results from a disorder within the external or middle ear and affects air conduction, with preserved bone conduction on audiometry. SNHL affects both air and bone conduction and implies involvement of the otic capsule or cochlear nerve.

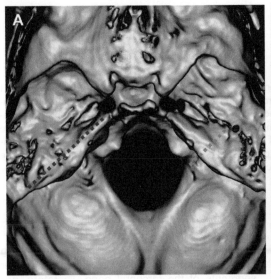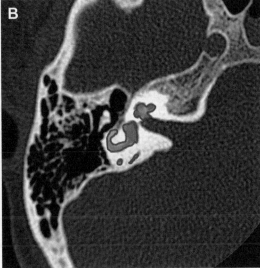

Fig. 2. Classification of temporal bone fractures. Three-dimensional (3D) volume -rendered CT image of the skull base (*A*) shows the trajectory of a longitudinal fracture of the right temporal bone (*A, red dashed line*) and a transverse fracture of the left temporal bone (*A, blue dashed line*). A fracture is categorized as mixed if both transverse and longitudinal fracture planes are present. Axial CT image of the temporal bone in a normal patient shows the normal anatomy of the bony labyrinth (*B*). An otic capsule–violating fracture may involve the cochlea, vestibule, semicircular canals, or vestibular aqueduct (*B, outlined in blue*).

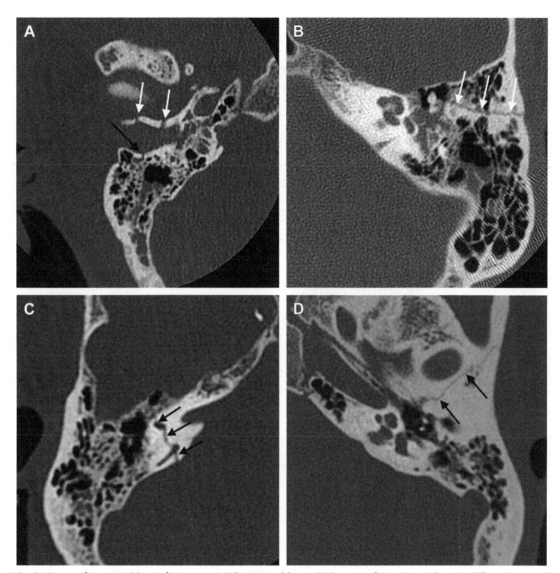

Fig. 3. Types of temporal bone fractures. Axial temporal bone CT images of 4 patients show 4 different types of temporal bone fractures (*A–D*). (*A*) A segmental longitudinal fracture of the tympanic ring (*A, white arrows*) with an additional fracture that extends through the mastoid (*A, black arrow*) with associated hemorrhage in the external auditory canal. (*B*) A characteristic longitudinal extralabyrinthine fracture of the mastoid that extends into the middle ear cavity (*B, white arrows*). (*C*) A transverse intralabyrinthine fracture with involvement of the semicircular canals (*C, black arrows*). (*D*) A transverse extralabyrinthine fracture traversing the squamous portion of the temporal bone (*D, black arrows*).

CHL

Traumatic CHL can occur from tympanic membrane perforation, hemotympanum, and derangement of the ossicular chain. In a review of 699 patients with 820 temporal bone fractures, Brodie and Thompson[4] reported that 21% of patients with hearing loss had a conductive type. CHL was identified in 80% of patients with hearing loss in the study by Dahiya and colleagues.[1] The most common cause of transient mild CHL is related to the presence of hemotympanum and tympanic membrane perforation.[13] A persistent CHL, defined as an air-bone gap measuring greater than 30 dB for longer than 6 weeks, usually implies a more significant injury and should raise concern for ossicular injury.[14]

Ossicular Injury

Ossicular injury may be related to direct traumatic forces or indirectly related to simultaneous tetanic contraction of the stapedius and tensor tympani muscles.[13,15] Injury to the ossicular chain occurs

Table 2
Summary of temporal bone fracture classification literature

Investigators, Date	Study Design	Results	Conclusions
Ghorayeb & Yeakley,[5] 1992	Evaluated direction classification and incorporated the oblique descriptor into the classification scheme	150 fractures in 140 pts • 112 (74.7%) oblique • 4 (2.7%) longitudinal • 18 (12%) transverse • 14 (9.3%) mixed • 2 (1.3%) petrous apex	Most fractures are more complex than traditional classification suggests. Most fractures are oblique, crossing the petrotympanic fissure

Brodie & Thompson,[4] 1997	Reviewed incidence of complications from temporal bone fractures. Incorporated otic capsule–sparing vs otic capsule–violating terminology; all otic capsule–violating fractures were classified as transverse fractures	820 fractures in 699 pts
		• 799 (97.5%) OCS
		  ○ 6% FN injury
		  ○ 16% CSF fistula
		• 21 (2.5%) OCV
		  ○ 48% FN injury
		  ○ 31% CSF fistula
			OCS fractures were most common. FN injury and CSF fistula were common in OCV injuries. CSF fistulae typically resolve spontaneously but, if persistent, pts are at risk for developing meningitis

Dahiya et al,[1] 1999	Compared traditional classification with otic capsule–sparing/ violating fractures and assessed associated complications	55 fractures
		• 21 (38%) longitudinal
		• 34 (62%) mixed/oblique
		• 50 (94%) OCS
		• 5 (6%) OCV
		  ○ 2-fold increase in FN injury
		  ○ 4-fold increase in CSF leak
		  ○ 7-fold increase in SNHL
			Temporal bone fractures should be classified based on whether the otic capsule is violated or intact. OCV fractures have a high association with FN injury, CSF leak, and SNHL

Ishman & Friedland,[8] 2004	Compared traditional classification with petrous vs nonpetrous fracture classification and assessed associated complications	155 fractures in 132 pts
		• 99 (64%) longitudinal
		  ○ 4% CSF leak
		  ○ 4% FN injury
		  ○ 46% CHL
		• 36 (23%) transverse
		  ○ 6% CSF leak
		  ○ 14% FN injury
		  ○ 62% CHL
		• 20 (13%) mixed
		  ○ 25% CSF leak
		  ○ 25% FN injury
		  ○ 50% CHL
		• 154 (99.4%) nonpetrous
		  ○ 4% CSF leak
		  ○ 7% FN injury
		  ○ 56% CHL
		• 18 (12%) petrous
		  ○ 33% CSF leak
		  ○ 22% FN injury
		  ○ 20% CHL
			There is poor correlation between traditional classification systems and complications related to temporal bone fracture. Investigators advocate an anatomy-based classification system. Fractures that involve the petrous portion of the temporal bone had the highest association with FN injury and CSF leak. Nonpetrous fractures had the greatest correlation with CHL

(continued on next page)

Table 2
(continued)

Investigators, Date	Study Design	Results	Conclusions

Rafferty et al,[11] 2006	Compared traditional and otic capsule classification systems and assessed associated complications	31 pts
		• 9 (29%) longitudinal
		  ○ 0% SNHL
		• 8 (26%) horizontal
		  ○ 50% SNHL
		• 14 (45%) mixed
		• 29 (93%) otic capsule–sparing
		  ○ 3% CSF leak
		  ○ 7% SNHL
		  ○ 52% brain injury
		• 2 (7%) otic capsule violating
		  ○ 50% CSF leak
		  ○ 100% SNHL
		  ○ 100% brain injury
			Neither classification system was superior in anticipating associated complications. Investigators recognized that the small sample size may have diminished the power of their study

Little & Kesser,[6] 2008	Compared traditional and otic capsule classification systems and assessed associated complications	30 pts
		• 15 (50%) longitudinal
		• 8 (25%) transverse
		• 7 (23%) oblique
		• 24 (80%) otic capsule–sparing
		  ○ 13% FN injury
		  ○ 4% SNHL
		• 6 (20%) otic capsule violating
		  ○ 67% FN injury
		  ○ 100% SNHL
			OCV fractures had a stronger correlation with FN injury and SNHL than OCS fractures. There was no significant difference in complication rate between fractures based on direction

Abbreviations: FN, facial nerve; OCS, otic capsule sparing; OCV, otic capsule violating; pts, patients.

more often with longitudinally oriented fractures that extend into the middle ear than with transverse-type fractures.[7,16,17] Ossicular injuries include fractures of the ossicles as well as dislocation of the incudomalleolar joint, incudostapedial joint, malleoincudal complex, incus, stapediovestibular joint, and the suspensory ligaments of the ossicles (**Figs. 4–10**).[16,17] Patients with ossicular derangement often sustain more than one type of ossicular injury.[17] The incus is the ossicle most commonly affected in the setting of temporal bone trauma because of its large size and weak ligamentous support within the tympanic cavity (see **Figs. 6** and **7**).[13] However, there is some debate about which joint is most often affected. Some studies report a higher incidence of incudomalleolar joint dislocation (see **Fig. 4**) and others report a higher incidence of incudostapedial dislocation (see **Fig. 5**).[7,13,16–18] Basson and van Lierop[13] reported a 63% occurrence of incudostapedial joint dislocation in their small review of 16 patients. In contrast, Meriot and colleagues[16] identified a higher percentage of incudomalleolar joint dislocation compared with incudostapedial

involvement in their larger retrospective review of 163 patients.

Imaging of ossicular injury

The ossicular joints may be described as subluxed if there is only mild separation of the ossicles, and dislocated if there is frank separation of the ossicles (see **Figs. 4** and **5**). The incudomalleolar joint has a characteristic appearance on axial images with an ice-cream-cone configuration; the head of the malleus representing the ice cream and the incus representing the cone (see **Fig. 4A**). Derangement of the incudomalleolar joint is easily assessed on axial CT images even in the setting of associated hemotympanum (see **Figs. 4** and **6–8**). Coronal or oblique reconstructions may provide an additional perspective on ossicular malalignment (see **Fig. 4D**).[19]

The integrity of the incudostapedial joint is often more difficult to assess in the setting of trauma because hemotympanum typically obscures this small anatomic structure. The incudostapedial joint can be evaluated by scrolling through a series of axial CT images and assessing the relative

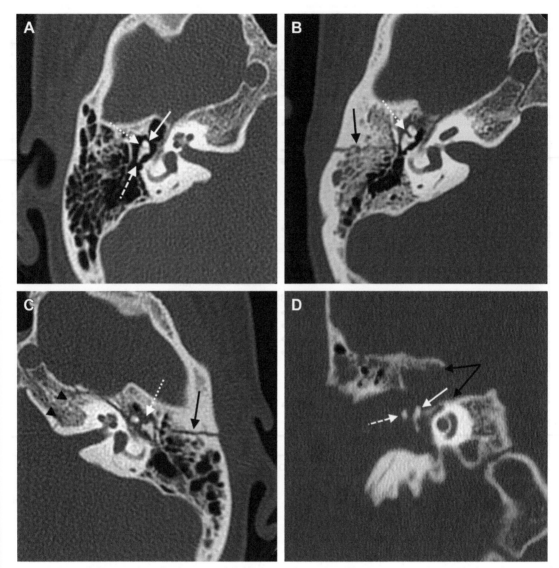

Fig. 4. Injury of the incudomalleolar joint. (*A*) The normal incudomalleolar joint in the axial plane (*A, dotted arrow*) with the head of the malleus (*A, solid arrow*) in close apposition with the body of the incus (*dashed arrow*). Disruption of the incudomalleolar joint can be easily identified in the axial and coronal planes and is shown in these 3 examples (*C, D*). (*B*) Mild subluxation of the incudomalleolar joint space (*B, dotted arrow*) related to an extralabyrinthine longitudinal fracture (*B, solid arrow*). (*C*) Frank dislocation of the incudomalleolar joint (*C, dotted arrow*) related to an extralabyrinthine longitudinal fracture (*B, solid arrow*). A transverse fracture of the petrous temporal bone is also present in this patient (*C, arrowheads*). Dislocation of the incudomalleolar joint can be seen in the coronal plane and has been described as the Y sign (*D*).[19] (*D*) There is lateralization of the incus (*D, dashed white arrow*) with respect to the malleus (*D, solid white arrow*) with an intervening gap. Also note the wide fracture gap through the tegmen (*D, solid black arrows*).

position of the long and lenticular processes of the incus with the capitellum, crura, and footplate of the stapes (see **Fig. 5**). Total incus dislocation can occur if the incus is dislocated at both the incudomalleolar and incudostapedial joints (see **Figs. 6** and **7**). In addition, the malleus and incus may be dislocated as a unit with primary disarticulation of the incudostapedial joint (see **Fig. 5**C).

Disruption of the stapediovestibular joint is rare, being reported in only 3% of cases, likely because of its strong attachment by the annular ligament.[16]

Ossicular fractures are also infrequent, occurring in approximately 2% to 11% of cases.[7,16] Some studies report the stapes and others report the incus as the most commonly fractured ossicle.[16,17] Stapes fractures may involve the

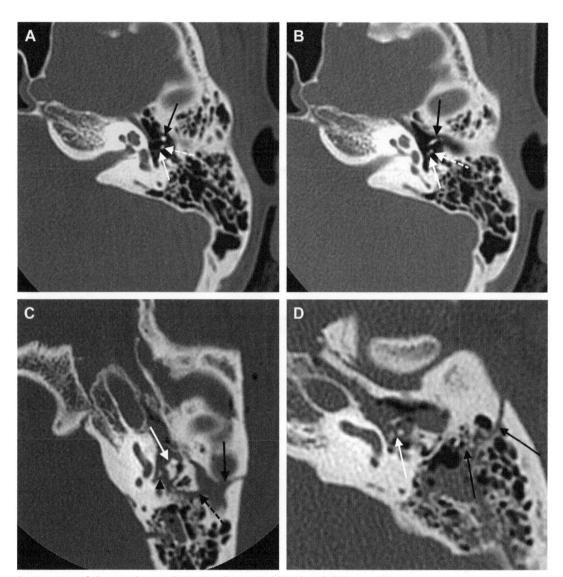

Fig. 5. Injury of the incudostapedial joint. The normal (*A*, *B*) and dislocated (*C*, *D*) appearance of the incudosta-pedial joint in the axial plane. At the level of the oval window, the normal appearance of the stapes is well pro-filed (*A*, *solid white arrow*) with visualization of the anterior and posterior crura. The distal tip of the long process of the incus is seen at this level (*A*, *dashed white arrow*) and the malleus is seen anteriorly (*black arrow*). Just below the oval window (*B*), the incudostapedial joint is profiled, showing the close apposition between the lenticular process of the incus (*B*, *dashed arrow*) and the capitellum of the stapes (*B*, *solid white arrow*). The malleus is anterior to the incudostapedial joint (*B*, *black arrow*). (*C*) Frank dislocation of the incudostapedial joint showing anterior and inferior dislocation of incudomalleolar complex (*C*, *white arrow*), which is now at the level of the stapes superstructure (*C*, *black arrowhead*). These findings are related to a displaced fracture fragment (*C*, *dashed black arrow*) from an extralabyrinthine oblique fracture (*B*, *solid black arrow*). (*D*) Mild subluxation of the incudostapedial joint in a different patient shown by mild widening of the joint space (*D*, *white arrow*) related to an underlying oblique temporal bone fracture (*D*, *black arrows*).

capitellum, arch, or footplate. Footplate fractures (see **Fig. 10**) are often related to transverse frac-tures, which extend through the oval window, whereas fractures of the arch most commonly occur in the setting of torsional forces.[16] Perilym-phatic fistula (PLF) should be suspected in those patients with fractures that traverse the footplate. Axial CT images are most useful in the assessment of ossicular fractures, which can be subtle on imaging. The presence of a lucent line through the ossicles as well as a displaced bone fragment should raise the suspicion for an ossicular fracture

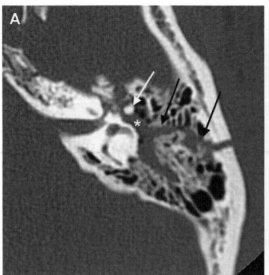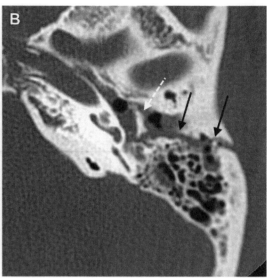

Fig. 6. Total incus dislocation. Axial CT images of the left temporal bone (A, B) show absence of the incus from its normal position within the incudal fossa (A, asterisk) with preservation of the normal position of the malleus (A, white arrow) related to a longitudinal extralabyrinthine fracture (A, B, black arrows). The incus is rotated and inferiorly positioned within the tympanic cavity (B, dashed arrow).

(see Fig. 9). Coronal reconstructions may better evaluate fractures of the manubrium and long process of the incus because of the vertical orientation of these ossicles (see Fig. 9).

Treatment of ossicular injury

Several treatment strategies have been used to manage patients with posttraumatic CHL, ranging from immediate exploration to delayed repair after 3 to 6 months. A conservative approach is likely warranted in those patients with tympanic membrane perforation, hemotympanum, and minor ossicular derangements because many of these patient's symptoms resolve without intervention. In a review of 45 patients presenting with posttraumatic CHL, Grant and colleagues[20] identified that 77% of ears showed improvement in pure tone averages using a conservative approach and only 5 of 47 ears eventually required surgical management. Surgery may be indicated in those patients with persistent CHL for longer than 6 months. Surgical repair of ossicular chain incongruencies is intended to restore transmission of sound from the tympanic membrane to the oval window and can be achieved using bone, cartilage, or prosthetic grafts depending on the location and type of ossicular injury. Reconstruction of the ossicular chain was performed in 5 patients in the study by Brodie and Thompson[4] with an average postoperative air-bone gap of 17.5 dB. Postsurgical improvement in CHL was also noted in 4 of 5 patients in the series by Dahiya and colleagues.[1]

SNHL

Traumatic SNHL may be caused by fractures that involve the labyrinth (see Fig. 10; Fig. 11) or internal auditory canal as well as by isolated intralabyrinthine hemorrhage without fracture (Fig. 12). In the past, transverse -type fractures have been reported to have a stronger correlation with SNHL. However, newer classification schemes that compare traditional classification methods with otic capsule–sparing/violating schemes argue that directional classification schemes are less predictive of complications including SNHL.[1,6,11] Otic capsule–violating fractures, which represent 2% to 6% of temporal bone fractures, are invariably associated with profound SNHL.[1,4,6] One study reports that otic capsule–violating fractures are 25 times more likely to be associated with SNHL than if the otic capsule is spared.[6] However, patients classified into the more traditional transverse, longitudinal, and oblique fracture patterns had similar percentages of SNHL, showing the lack of specificity of the directional classification scheme in predicting posttraumatic SNHL.[6]

Axial CT images are optimal at identifying otic capsule–violating fractures as manifested by fracture lines that extend through the cochlea, vestibule, or semicircular canal (see Figs. 1C, 3C, 10, and 11). Pneumolabyrinth may be seen as a secondary sign indicating that the otic capsule has been violated (see Figs. 1C and 10). Identifying hemorrhage within the otic capsule is not possible on CT. Magnetic resonance (MR) imaging may

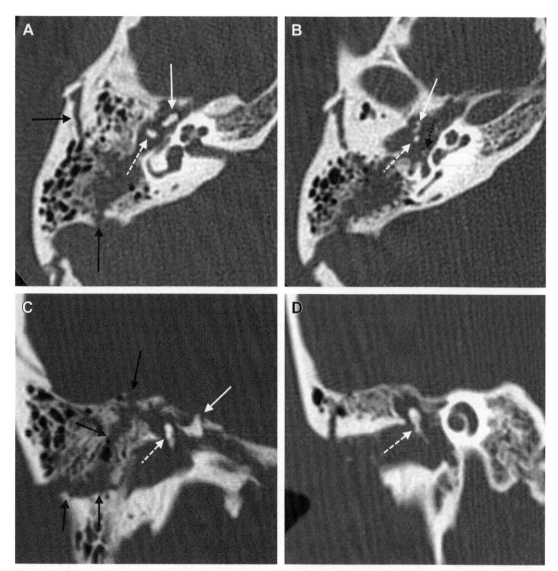

Fig. 7. Total incus dislocation. Axial and Stenvers reconstructions of the right temporal bone (*A–D*) show total incus dislocation related to a complex temporal bone fracture (*black arrows*). The incus is rotated with anterior and superior displacement (*white solid arrows*). Note the superior displacement of incus through the fractured tegmen on the Stenvers reconstruction (*C, solid white arrow*). The malleus (*white dashed arrows*) and stapes (*B, black dashed arrow*) remain normal in position.

show evidence of hemolabyrinth in some patients with trauma with SNHL even in the absence of fracture (see **Fig. 12**).

Vertigo

Patients may also experience vertigo, dizziness, or disequilibrium following temporal bone trauma.[21] As in SNHL, vertigo may result from fracture that violates the vestibule, semicircular canals, vestibular aqueduct, or vestibular nerve. In the absence of fracture, patients may have vertigo from a labyrinthine concussion, shearing of the nerve root entry zone, or from brainstem injury.[12,21] Alternate diagnoses including PLF and otolith dislocation should also be entertained in patients with vertigo without associated fracture.[12] Posttraumatic vertigo typically resolves spontaneously after 6 to 12 months.[12]

Axial CT images remain best for evaluating the labyrinth for associated fractures that violate the vestibular apparatus (see **Figs. 1**C, **3**C, **10**, and **11**). Stenvers and Pöschl reconstructions may be beneficial additional views because they profile the posterior and superior semicircular canals respectively. An MR examination using a gradient

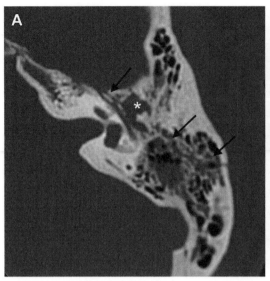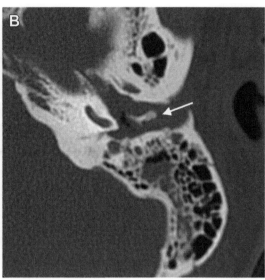

Fig. 8. Malleus dislocation. Axial CT images of the left temporal bone show malleus dislocation (*A, B*) related to a longitudinal otic capsule–sparing fracture (*black arrows*). The malleus is externally rotated and inferiorly dislocated (*B, white arrow*) from its normal position within the tympanic cavity (*A, asterisk*).

echo sequence may reveal hemorrhage within the vestibular nucleus or nerve root entry zone within the brainstem in patients with persistent vertiginous symptoms without a clear underlying cause on CT.

PLF

PLFs result from an abnormal connection between the perilymph and middle ear cavity and can be

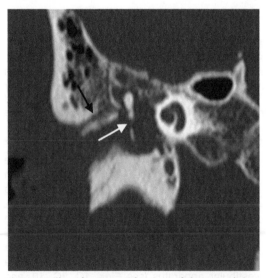

Fig. 9. Malleus fracture. A fracture of the manubrium of the malleus with inferior positioning of the lower fracture fragment (*white arrow*) related to a longitudinal otic capsule–sparing temporal bone fracture (*black arrow*).

traumatic, congenital, or spontaneous.[22] Posttraumatic PLFs allow perilymph to leak into the tympanic cavity and may be related to disruption of the oval window or, less commonly, of the round window membrane.[21] Traumatic PLFs may occur from implosive or explosive mechanisms as described by Goodhill[23] in 1971. Direct external trauma to the tympanic membrane, oval window, or round window may result in an implosive injury,[23] or a sudden increase in intracranial pressure transmitted through the perilymph to the oval or round window may result in an explosive PLF.[23] Patients with PLF may present with a confusing clinical picture including persistent vertigo with intermittent SNHL and/or CHL.[22] Symptoms of PLF typically begin within 24 to 72 hours after injury, which can be used as a feature distinguishing PLF from traumatic Meniere syndrome, which often occurs months to years after injury.[21,24]

Fractures through the stapes footplate or round window seen on CT should raise the suspicion of PLF (see **Fig. 10**). However, in the absence of a fracture, PLF is a difficult diagnosis to make. Pneumolabyrinth and unexplained dependently layering fluid within the middle ear may be secondary signs of PLF in patients without a temporal bone fracture.[22,24]

CSF Leak

Patients who sustain temporal bone injury are at risk for developing a CSF leak, a serious complication given the associated risk of meningitis. CSF leak may occur when there is violation of the skull

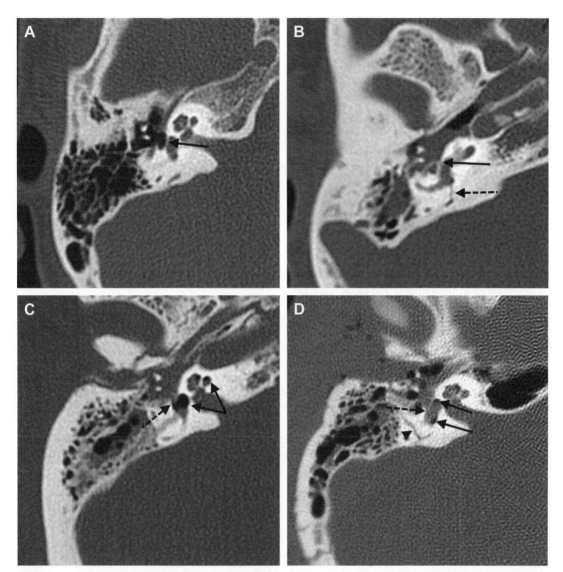

Fig. 10. Stapes footplate fractures. Axial CT images of the right temporal bone in 4 patients show the normal (*A*) and fractured appearance (*B–D*) of the stapes footplate. (*A*) The normal appearance of the stapes footplate and oval window in the axial plane (*A, arrow*). (*B*) A transverse otic capsule–violating fracture of the right temporal bone (*B, dashed arrow*). The fracture extends through the anterior margin of the stapes footplate (*B, solid arrow*). (*C*) A subtle depressed fracture of the stapes footplate (*C, dashed arrow*) with extensive associated pneumolabyrinth in the cochlea and vestibule (*C, solid arrows*). Although the fracture is subtle, the presence of air within the otic capsule should raise the suspicion for injury. (*D*) Another example of a subtle stapes footplate fracture (*D, dashed arrow*) with associated subtle pneumolabyrinth (*D, solid arrows*). An additional transverse fracture is identified coursing through the vestibular aqueduct (*D, arrowheads*). Fractures of the footplate should raise the concern for associated perilymphatic fistula.

and underlying dura. When CSF leaks involve the temporal bone, they can present as otorrhea with a disrupted tympanic membrane, or otorhinorrhea with an intact tympanic membrane via eustachian tube drainage.[25] A high index of suspicion is required for appropriate management of these patients because CSF leaks may be clinically subtle and related to slow, often positional, leakage of fluid. Confirmatory beta-2 transferrin testing should be performed for those patients in whom CSF leak is suspected.[25]

Posttraumatic CSF leak has been reported to occur in 13% to 45% of patients with temporal bone fractures, with meningitis in 7% of patients.[1,4,7,8,11] The risk of developing meningitis in the setting of CSF leak is multifactorial, the most

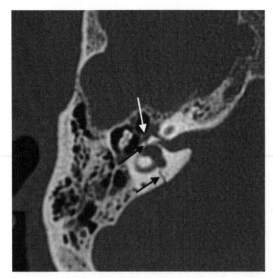

Fig. 11. Fracture of the vestibule and facial nerve canal. Axial CT image of the right temporal bone shows a transverse otic capsule–violating fracture that extends through the vestibule (*black arrows*), which propagates through the tympanic segment of the facial nerve canal (*white arrow*).

significant risk being related to the duration of CSF leak.[4] Patients with CSF leaks that continue for longer than 7 days are at higher risk of developing meningitis compared with those patients whose leaks stop by day 7.[4] It is rare for meningitis to

occur in the absence of a CSF leak, therefore prophylactic antibiotic therapy is indicated only in those patients with a CSF leak. Patients with trauma who sustain injury to the temporal bone may have multiple skull base fractures, with alternate sources of CSF leak outside the temporal bone. Therefore precise localization of the site of CSF leak is critical in managing these patients with skull base trauma, because the surgical approach may be different depending on the anatomic location of the leak. There is an association between fracture pattern and the development of CSF leak. Patients with otic capsule–violating fractures are 4 to 8 times more likely to have a CSF leak than patients with otic capsule–sparing fractures.[1,4,6] However, the traditional directional classification scheme is a poor predictor of the presence or absence of CSF leak.[6,11]

Imaging findings of CSF leak
Scrutinizing the integrity and position of the tegmen is critical when evaluating temporal bone CT scans for potential sites of posttraumatic CSF leaks. Coronal and sagittal reconstructions are best at evaluating the tegmen for defects (**Fig. 13**). It is important to describe the location and size of the fracture defect, the presence and orientation of displaced fracture fragments through the defect, and the presence of any associated encephalocele (see **Fig. 13**). In the authors'

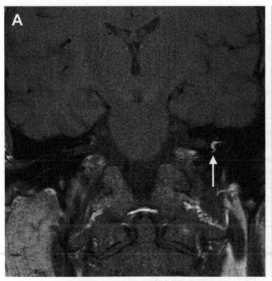
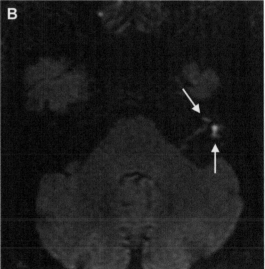

Fig. 12. Intralabyrinthine hemorrhage without fracture. Coronal unenhanced T1 (*A*) and axial T2 fluid-attenuated inversion recovery (FLAIR) (*B*) images through the internal auditory canals in a patient who presented with hearing loss after a minor fall shows findings of hemolabyrinth. There is intrinsic T1 signal hyperintensity (*A, arrow*) and T2-FLAIR signal hyperintensity (*B, arrows*) within the semicircular canals, vestibule, and cochlea of the left temporal bone. A head CT scan performed initially showed no evidence of temporal bone fracture or other abnormality within the brain (not shown).

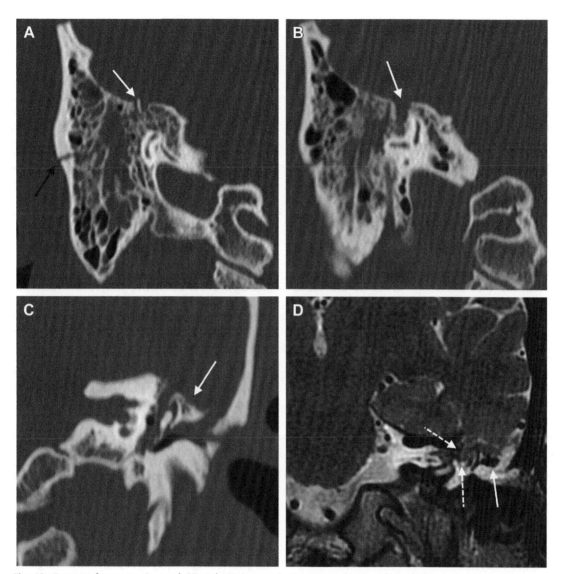

Fig. 13. Tegmen fractures. Coronal CT and MR images in 2 patients (*A, B* and *C, D*) show examples of fractures through the tegmen with associated complications. Coronal CT images of the right temporal bone (*A, B*) show an oblique fracture that involves the mastoid (*A, black arrow*) that extends through the tegmen with an associated fracture gap (*B, white arrow*). There is a fracture fragment that is perpendicular to the dura (*A, white arrow*) which may act as a wick, increasing the risk of subsequent CSF leak. Coronal CT and MR imaging of the left temporal bone in a different patient (*C, D*) shows a large defect within the left tegmen with an associated displaced fracture fragment (*C, D, solid white arrow*). There is evidence of a posttraumatic encephalocele with herniation of brain tissue and CSF through the fracture gap, which is seen best on MR (*D, dashed arrows*).

experience, factors that may increase the risk of persistent posttraumatic CSF leak include a widely spaced fracture defect and the presence of a bone spicule oriented perpendicular to the dura potentially acting as a wick (see **Figs. 4**D, **7**C, and **13**). Patients with persistent symptoms of CSF leak beyond 7 to 10 days may require further evaluation with MR imaging. MR imaging of the brain with dedicated high-resolution T2-weighted sequences of the temporal bone may be complementary to CT in evaluating patients specifically for the location and size of associated encephaloceles (see **Fig. 13**D). Contrast is indicated in these patients because the presence of dural enhancement may be a secondary sign of a dural tear, CSF leak, and focal meningitis.

Treatment of CSF leak

Most posttraumatic CSF leaks (78% in one series) resolve spontaneously within 7 days of injury.[4]

Therefore a conservative approach including bed rest with an elevated head, decreased straining, and lumbar drain is often warranted in these patients until day 10.[4] Surgical closure in those patients with persistent CSF leaks beyond day 10 is often performed because of the increased risk of meningitis.[4] The surgical approach for the treatment of CSF leaks depends on several factors including location of the leak, ipsilateral and contralateral hearing status, presence of associated encephalocele, and integrity of the external canal.[4] In patients whose hearing is completely compromised in the ipsilateral ear, a more aggressive approach is taken with obliteration of the middle ear and mastoid with placement of a duroplasty. Less aggressive approaches may be indicated in patients with intact hearing, including transmastoid, middle fossa, and combined approaches with placement of temporalis fascia over the defect.[4,26]

Facial Nerve Injury

The facial nerve's circuitous course through the temporal bone places it at risk for injury in multiple locations in the setting of temporal bone fracture. However, detectable injury to the facial nerve remains rare, occurring in an estimated 5% to 10% of patients with temporal bone fractures.[4,17,27] Motor vehicle accidents are implicated in 44% to 54% of cases of traumatic facial nerve palsy, followed by falls and assaults. The reported risk of facial palsy associated with temporal bone fracture has been gradually decreasing, likely because of increasing rates of seat belt use, the development of airbag technology, and increasing recognition of subtle temporal bone fractures though the use of CT.[21]

In the past, facial nerve palsy has had a greater association with transverse fractures than with the more common longitudinal temporal bone fracture.[28] Fractures that involve the otic capsule are similarly more likely to be associated with facial nerve paralysis than those that spare the otic capsule (48 vs 6%).[4] However, because otic capsule–sparing fractures are between 5 and 40 times more frequent than those involving the otic capsule, most trauma-related facial nerve palsy cases are caused by otic capsule–sparing fractures.[1,4,6]

Injury to the facial nerve can be caused by compression, contusion, stretching, perineural or intraneural hematoma, and/or nerve transection.[29] These injury patterns are typically inferred on CT because of displacement or violation of the facial canal (Fig. 14). High-resolution MR imaging of the temporal bone can directly show perineural hematomas, particularly those of the geniculate ganglion. MR imaging also allows demonstration of abnormal contrast enhancement in segments affected by scarring or fibrosis.[30]

The geniculate ganglion is consistently reported to be the most common site of injury of the facial nerve, implicated in 30% to 80% of cases of facial nerve paresis (see Fig. 14B). Other sites, including the canalicular, labyrinthine, tympanic, and mastoid segments, are less commonly involved (see Figs. 11 and 14).[22,28] Lambert and Brackman[28] identified synchronous lesions in the mastoid segment in 15% of patients in their series, suggesting that multiple sites of injury should be considered, particularly in patients with complex or comminuted fractures.

Treatment of facial nerve injury

Management of facial nerve palsy related to temporal bone fractures is controversial, with guidelines largely based on retrospective case series and established clinical practice.[27] Patients with delayed-onset facial palsy have an excellent prognosis, with greater than 90% eventually regaining House-Brackman (HB) grade I or II facial nerve function without surgical intervention. Patients with incomplete paresis (<90% of loss of function on electroneurography) also have a high rate of recovery, with large series reporting nearly universal recovery to HB grade I or II facial nerve function.[4,21,27]

Surgical management is typically limited to those patients with complete, immediate facial nerve paralysis and those with progressive near-complete loss of function.[31] The goals of surgery are to evaluate and decompress the facial nerve, with the addition of nerve rerouting, reanastomosis, or sural nerve grafting as indicated based on surgical findings. Injury at or proximal to the geniculate ganglion may require a middle fossa or transmastoid/supralabyrinthine approach in patients with intact hearing. For those patients with complete hearing loss, a translabyrinthine approach is possible and allows excellent exposure of the facial nerve. Exposure of the more distal tympanic and mastoid segments is typically achieved through a transmastoid approach.[4,23,31]

In surgical candidates with immediate, complete facial nerve paralysis there is a high rate of return of facial nerve function following decompression, with good (HB I or II) recovery in 38% to 55% of patients. In a recent meta-analysis of 612 patients with facial nerve paresis, only 6% of patients who were surgically decompressed showed persistent complete (HB VI) facial palsy.[27] Poor prognostic indicators for incomplete regrowth of the facial nerve include bone spicules that occlude the facial canal and widely displaced canal margins.

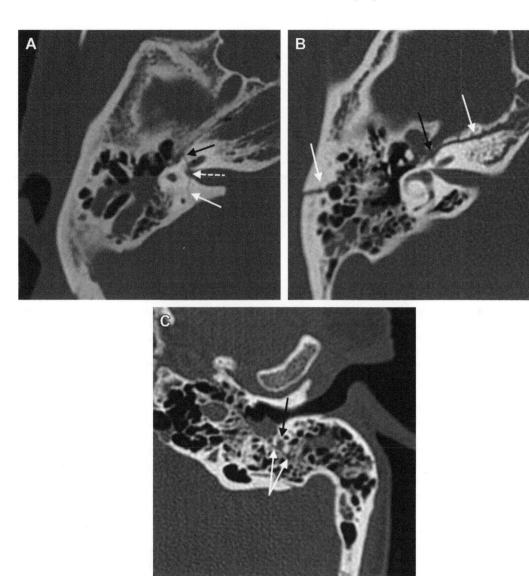

Fig. 14. Injury of the facial nerve canal. Axial CT images of 3 patients show fractures that violate the facial nerve canal (A–C). (A) A transverse intralabyrinthine fracture (A, *solid white arrow*) that extends through the fundus of the internal auditory canal (A, *dashed white arrow*) and subsequently propagates through the tympanic segment of the facial nerve canal (A, *black arrow*). (B) An otic capsule–sparing longitudinal fracture (B, *white arrows*) that extends through the mastoid, middle ear cavity, geniculate fossa of the facial nerve (B, *black arrow*), and through the petrous apex. (C) A nondisplaced longitudinal fracture of the left mastoid (C, *white arrows*) that extends through the medial aspect of the mastoid segment of the facial nerve canal (C, *black arrow*).

Timing of surgical decompression, when indicated, is also controversial. Some clinicians advocate decompression within 72 hours, which can be difficult to achieve in patients with multiple injuries, or those who initially present to centers that lack the surgical expertise to perform immediate decompression. There is evidence that surgical decompression within 2 weeks has the best probability (>90%) of a good outcome, with gradual diminution in prognosis for decompression performed up to and past 3 months.[22] However, even delayed decompression at 2 to 3 months may result in a good outcome in more than 50% of patients. Delayed decompression can be helpful in those whose injuries masked initial signs of facial paralysis, or those with a delayed presentation to a center with experience in facial nerve decompression.[21,22,29]

Vascular Injury

The carotid artery and venous vascular structures that traverse the temporal bone are at risk for injury in the setting of temporal bone trauma. The carotid artery enters the skull base through the carotid

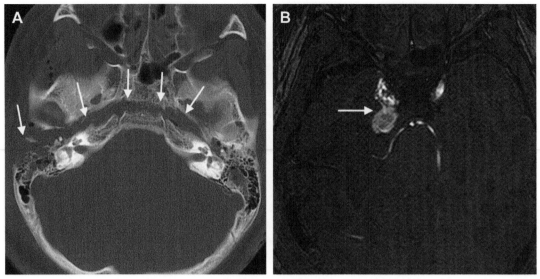

Fig. 15. Carotid canal injury. Axial head CT (*A*) of a patient involved in a skiing accident shows an extensive displaced fracture of the petrous portion of the right temporal bone and central skull base with widely separated fracture margins (*A*, *white arrows*). The fracture courses through the bilateral petrous carotid canals. 3D time-of-flight MR angiography of the circle of Willis (*B*) shows arterialized flow within the right cavernous sinus with a large associated outpouching that indicates a traumatic cavernous carotid fistula with pseudoaneurysm formation (*B*, *white arrow*).

canal and passes through the petrous portion of the temporal bone before it ascends within the cavernous sinus. In one series, carotid canal involvement was seen in 24% of patients with skull base fractures.[32] Resnick and colleagues[32] noted that 11% of patients with skull base fractures that involved the carotid canal showed evidence of vascular injury. Therefore fractures that extend through the carotid canal should be further evaluated with either CT angiography or MR angiography to assess for associated vascular complications including dissection, transection, pseudoaneurysm formation, occlusion, and arteriovenous fistula (Fig. 15).

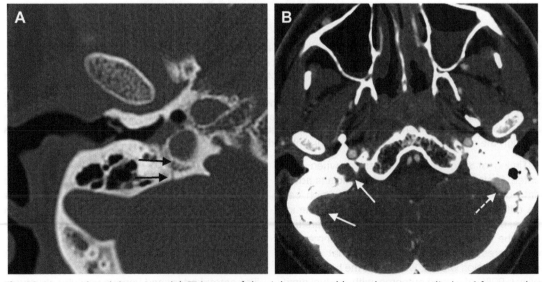

Fig. 16. Venous sinus injury. An axial CT image of the right temporal bone shows a nondisplaced fracture that extends into the jugular foramen (*A*, *arrows*). A postcontrast CT venogram shows nonpacification of the right sigmoid sinus and jugular bulb (*B*, *solid arrows*) indicating thrombus related to traumatic venous sinus injury. Note the normal contrast-enhanced appearance of the left sigmoid sinus (*B*, *dashed arrow*).

The distal transverse and sigmoid sinuses travel through the posterior fossa within a groove along the medial margin of the mastoid portion of the temporal bone before exiting the skull base at the jugular foramen. These venous structures may also be injured when a fracture violates the sinodural plate or extends into the jugular foramen. It is important to review the soft tissue algorithm images of the posterior fossa as part of the temporal bone CT examination to assess for associated hyperdense venous sinus thrombosis, venous epidural hematoma, as well as associated cerebellar hemorrhage. Further evaluation with either CT venography or MR venography should be performed in those patients with fractures that involve the venous sinuses to assess the integrity of the venous system more comprehensively (**Fig. 16**).

SUMMARY

Temporal bone trauma is commonly seen in patients with craniofacial injury and can be detected using multidetector CT. A thorough understanding of the different types of temporal bone fracture patterns is needed to accurately describe the trajectory of injury as well as anticipated complications. Fractures should be described based on direction, segment of temporal bone involved, as well as involvement of the otic capsule. More importantly, the radiologist plays an integral role in identifying complications of temporal bone injury, which often have significant clinical implications.

REFERENCES

1. Dahiya R, Keller JD, Litofsky NS, et al. Temporal bone fractures: otic capsule sparing versus otic capsule violating clinical and radiographic considerations. J Trauma 1999;47(6):1079–83.
2. Exadaktylos AK, Sclabas GM, Nuyens M, et al. The clinical correlation of temporal bone fractures and spiral computed tomographic scan: a prospective and consecutive study at a level I trauma center. J Trauma 2003;55(4):704–6.
3. Alvi A, Bereliani AT. Trauma to the temporal bone: diagnosis and management of complications. J Craniomaxillofac Trauma 1996;2(3):36–48.
4. Brodie HA, Thompson TC. Management of complications from 820 temporal bone fractures. Am J Otolaryngol 1997;18(2):188–97.
5. Ghorayeb BY, Yeakley JW. Temporal bone fractures: longitudinal or oblique? The case for oblique temporal bone fractures. Laryngoscope 1992;102(2):129–34.
6. Little SC, Kesser BW. Radiographic classification of temporal bone fractures: clinical predictability using

a new system. Arch Otolaryngol Head Neck Surg 2006;132(12):1300–4.
7. Nosan DK, Benecke JE Jr, Murr AH. Current perspective on temporal bone trauma. Otolaryngol Head Neck Surg 1997;117(1):67–71.
8. Ishman SL, Friedland DR. Temporal bone fractures: traditional classification and clinical relevance. Laryngoscope 2004;114(10):1734–41.
9. Davidson HC. Imaging of the temporal bone. Neuroimaging Clin N Am 2004;14(4):721–60.
10. Gentry LR. Temporal bone trauma: current perspectives for diagnostic evaluation. Neuroimaging Clin N Am 1991;1:319–40.
11. Rafferty MA, Mc Conn Walsh R, Walsh MA. A comparison of temporal bone fracture classification systems. Clin Otolaryngol 2006;31(4):287–91.
12. Zayas JO, Feliciano YZ, Hadley CR, et al. Temporal bone trauma and the role of multidetector CT in the emergency department. Radiographics 2011;31(6):1741–55.
13. Basson OJ, van Lierop AC. Conductive hearing loss after head trauma: review of ossicular pathology, management and outcomes. J Laryngol Otol 2009;123(2):177–81.
14. Wennmo C, Spandow O. Fractures of the temporal bone–chain incongruencies. Am J Otolaryngol 1993;14(1):38–42.
15. Swartz JD. Temporal bone trauma. Semin Ultrasound CT MR 2001;22(3):219–28.
16. Meriot P, Veillon F, Garcia JF, et al. CT appearances of ossicular injuries. Radiographics 1997;17(6):1445–54.
17. Yetiser S, Hidir Y, Gonul E. Facial nerve problems and hearing loss in patients with temporal bone fractures: demographic data. J Trauma 2008;65(6):1314–20.
18. Bin Z, Jingzhen H, Daocai W, et al. Traumatic ossicular chain separation: sliding-thin-slab maximum-intensity projections for diagnosis. J Comput Assist Tomogr 2008;32(6):951–4.
19. Lourenco MT, Yeakley JW, Ghorayeb BY. The "Y" sign of lateral dislocation of the incus. Am J Otolaryngol 1995;16(3):387–92.
20. Grant JR, Arganbright J, Friedland DR. Outcomes for conservative management of traumatic conductive hearing loss. Otol Neurotol 2008;29(3):344–9.
21. Fitzgerald DC. Head trauma: hearing loss and dizziness. J Trauma 1996;40(3):488–96.
22. Swartz JD, Mukherji SK. The inner ear and otodystrophies. In: Swartz JD, Loevner LA, editors. Imaging of the temporal bone. 4th edition. New York: Thieme; 2009. p. 298–411.
23. Goodhill V. Sudden deafness and round window rupture. Laryngoscope 1971;81(9):1462–74.
24. Wang EY, Shatzkes D, Swartz JD. Temporal bone trauma. In: Swartz JD, Loevner LA, editors. Imaging of the temporal bone. New York: Thieme; 2009. p. 412–43.

25. Prosser JD, Vender JR, Solares CA. Traumatic cerebrospinal fluid leaks. Otolaryngol Clin North Am 2011;44(4):857–73, vii.

26. Oliaei S, Mahboubi H, Djalilian HR. Transmastoid approach to temporal bone cerebrospinal fluid leaks. Am J Otolaryngol 2012;33(5): 556–61.

27. Nash JJ, Friedland DR, Boorsma KJ, et al. Management and outcomes of facial paralysis from intratemporal blunt trauma: a systematic review. Laryngoscope 2010;120(7):1397–404.

28. Lambert PR, Brackmann DE. Facial paralysis in longitudinal temporal bone fractures: a review of 26 cases. Laryngoscope 1984;94(8):1022–6.

29. Ulug T, Arif Ulubil S. Management of facial paralysis in temporal bone fractures: a prospective study analyzing 11 operated fractures. Am J Otolaryngol 2005;26(4):230–8.

30. Sartoretti-Schefer S, Scherler M, Wichmann W, et al. Contrast-enhanced MR of the facial nerve in patients with posttraumatic peripheral facial nerve palsy. AJNR Am J Neuroradiol 1997;18(6):1115–25.

31. Patel A, Groppo E. Management of temporal bone trauma. Craniomaxillofac Trauma Reconstr 2010; 3(2):105–13.

32. Resnick DK, Subach BR, Marion DW. The significance of carotid canal involvement in basilar cranial fracture. Neurosurgery 1997;40(6):1177–81.

Cerebrovascular Trauma

Sara R. Nace, MD, Lindell R. Gentry, MD*

KEYWORDS

- Cerebrovascular • Trauma • Dissection • Diagnosis • Therapy

KEY POINTS

- Significant recent progress has been made in the recognition, screening, diagnosis, and treatment of blunt cerebrovascular injury (BCVI).
- Although controversy still exists as to optimal screening algorithms and best diagnostic modality, the vital and growing role of noninvasive imaging in identifying patients at high risk for BCVI and in characterizing the injury itself has been clearly established.
- There has been promising early work in stratifying BCVI patients into risk categories by initially evaluating them with high-resolution head, maxillofacial, and cervical computed tomographic (CT) examinations with the ultimate goal of maximizing diagnostic yield and enabling prompt initiation of therapy.
- Further work is needed to delineate the mechanistic relationship between craniofacial fractures and BCVI.
- Recent studies indicate the incidence of BCVI may be much higher (1%–3%) than initially reported (0.1%), due to the wider utilization of aggressive screening algorithms and noninvasive imaging.
- A high index of suspicion is necessary to identify BCVI, since many patients exhibit a latent, asymptomatic period.
- Untreated BCVI is associated with high morbidity and mortality. Identification and treatment of patients while they are asymptomatic has been shown to improve outcomes.
- CT angiography is the study of choice for initial imaging of traumatic CVI, although magnetic resonance imaging/magnetic resonance angiography demonstrates considerable value in characterizing vessel injury as well as associated ischemic complications.
- Current screening algorithms reinforce the importance of high-resolution head, maxillofacial, and cervical spine CT in identifying patients at high risk for BCVI.

INTRODUCTION

Historical Perspective and Significance of Traumatic Blunt Cerebrovascular Injury

The recognition of blunt cerebrovascular injury (BCVI) as an important diagnostic entity has occurred only in the past 2 decades, with continued current debate as to best practices in regards to screening, diagnosis, treatment, and follow-up.

The true incidence of BCVI in the setting of trauma is still not known but has been greatly underestimated in the past, largely because of a lack of routine imaging of asymptomatic patients. Before 1990, less than 200 total blunt carotid artery injury (BCAI) cases had been described in the literature.[1] Regionalization of trauma care caused these "uncommon" injuries to be funneled into fewer referral centers, generating greater interest in improving diagnosis. Many studies before the mid 1990s reported a 0.1% overall incidence of blunt injury to the carotid artery in trauma victims.[2–5] With subsequent utilization of aggressive screening criteria,

The authors have no disclosures.
Department of Radiology, University of Wisconsin, 600 Highland Avenue, Madison, WI 53792, USA
* Corresponding author.
E-mail address: lgentry@uwhealth.org

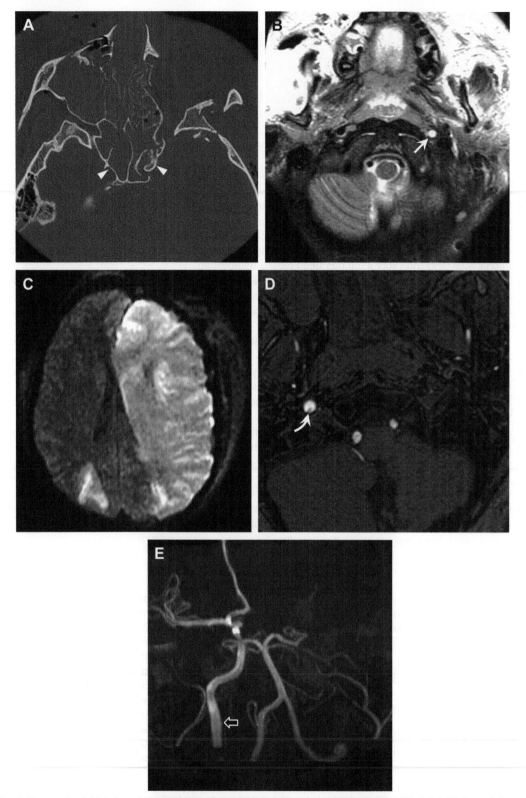

Fig. 1. Traumatic right internal carotid dissection and left internal carotid occlusion. (*A*) Axial CT shows bilateral fractures of the carotid canals (*arrowheads*) with more severe displacement on the left. (*B*) Axial T2-weighted and (*C*) diffusion-weighted MR images reveal a left carotid occlusion (*arrow*) and bilateral hemispheric infarcts, greater on the left. (*D*) 3D-TOF source and (*E*) maximum intensity projection (MIP) MRA images reveal a lack of flow in the left ICA and a dissection flap of the right ICA (*curved arrow*). The MIP image reveals slight overall enlargement of the distal right ICA (*open arrow*) but does not clearly reveal the dissection itself.

however, the incidence of documented cerebrovascular injury in blunt trauma patients increased 10-fold to 1%, and even higher (2.7%) when applied to patients with Injury Severity Scores of greater than or equal to 16.[1,6–11] Although initial emphasis was placed on carotid arterial injury (CAI), the incidence of vertebral artery injuries (VAI) from blunt trauma was found to range from 0.53% to 0.73%.[10,12]

Despite the relative infrequency of BCVI, devastating complications are very common in patients with documented injuries (Fig. 1). A 1998 review of the literature reported BCAI mortalities of 23%

to 28%, with even higher rates of permanent neurologic deficit (48%–58%).[7] Similarly, a mortality of 8% and permanent morbidity of 14% to 24% have been reported in untreated patients with blunt VAI.[10,12] Over the past decade, a growing body of evidence has revealed that a significant percentage of BCVI patients present in a delayed fashion, with ischemic events following a latent asymptomatic period. Antithrombotic medical therapy has been recently shown to decrease the incidence of posttraumatic stroke significantly and improve final neurologic outcome, emphasizing the importance of early diagnosis.[1,7,12,13]

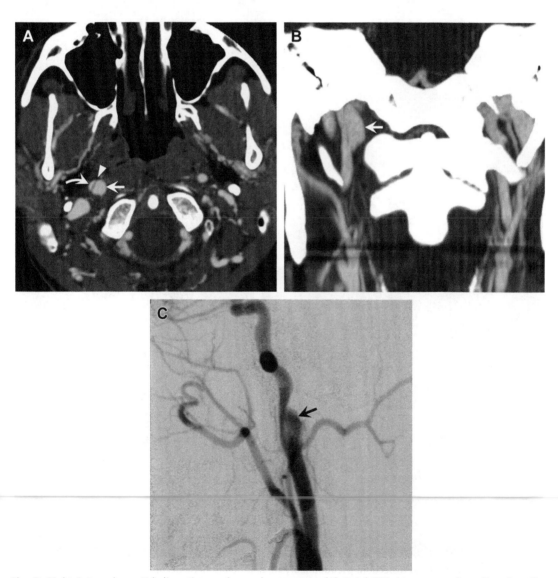

Fig. 2. Right internal carotid dissection and pseudoaneurysm. (A) Axial CTA image reveals a dissection flap (arrowhead) with a large pseudoaneurysm (arrow) that severely compresses the true ICA lumen (curved arrow). (B) Coronal 2D reconstructed CTA image and (C) lateral angiogram confirm the dissection, pseudoaneurysm (arrow), and compressed true ICA lumen.

As a result, aggressive screening protocols have been instituted, with an emphasis on utilization of noninvasive imaging modalities, such as computed tomographic angiography (CTA) and magnetic resonance angiography (MRA).

ANATOMY AND PATHOLOGY
Mechanisms and Patterns of Cerebrovascular Injury

Commonly accepted physiologic mechanisms of traumatic cerebrovascular injury include extreme cervical hyperextension/rotation, direct blunt vascular trauma, intraoral trauma, and direct laceration from bony fracture fragments.[14] Traumatic cerebrovascular dissections typically result from rapid deceleration of the body and resultant stretching of the involved vessel. This mechanism can be seen in patients following motor vehicle accidents, assault, pedestrian accidents, falls, and with hanging accidents.[7] Although consistently implicated as a risk factor for BCVI, the mechanisms associated with craniofacial fractures are not as well delineated.

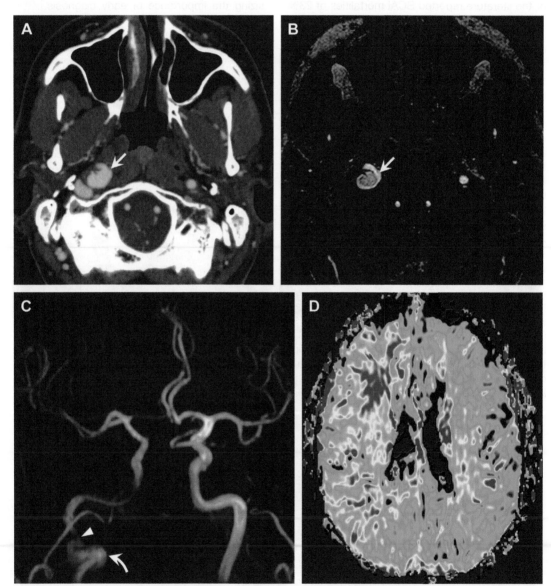

Fig. 3. Right internal carotid dissection, pseudoaneurysm, and hemispheric perfusion defect. (*A*) Axial CTA and (*B*) 3D-TOF MRA images reveal an enlarged, irregular ICA lumen compatible with traumatic pseudoaneurysm (*arrow*). (*C*) MIP MRA image confirms the pseudoaneurysm (*curved arrow*) and narrowed true ICA lumen (*arrowhead*). (*D*) Perfusion images demonstrate a prolonged transit time in the right hemisphere, indicating a risk of subsequent infarct.

The extracranial segments of the carotid and vertebral arteries are more vulnerable to traumatic injury than the intracranial segments because of their close relationship to surrounding osseous structures and relative greater mobility.[15,16] Extracranial carotid artery injuries most commonly occur in the distal cervical internal carotid artery (ICA) (**Figs. 2** and **3**). Injury is thought to result from stretching over the lateral masses of the cervical vertebrae (particularly C1-3) in the setting of head hyperextension and contralateral hyperrotation, and from impingement on the styloid process during head rotation. The ICA may also be compressed between the mandible or hyoid bone and the cervical spine during neck hyperflexion.[14–20] Prior studies have reported that superior displacement of the pterygoid plates (as in the case of Le Fort type fractures) poses a risk to the ICA inferior to the foramen lacerum.[21] Displaced bony fragments from skull base fractures may also lead to direct injury of the ICA.[14]

Extracranial VAI most commonly involves the V2 and V3 segments, because the vessel travels through the bony transverse foramina and around C1, respectively (**Figs. 4** and **5**).[22] Displaced fracture fragments of the cervical spine may directly lacerate these segments of the vertebral arteries.[14] Injuries to the V3 and V4 segments occur more commonly without associated cervical spine fracture/dislocation than injuries to the V2 segment.[23–25]

Although there is a relative dearth of data on incidence, it is generally accepted that intracranial cerebrovascular injury is less common than extracranial BCVI. Basilar skull fracture, certain patterns of facial fracture, and fractures extending through the carotid canal have been reported as risk factors for intracranial arterial injury (**Figs. 6** and **7**).[26] Manifestation of injury includes vascular compression, dissection, dissecting aneurysm, occlusion, arterial rupture, and arteriovenous fistula (carotid-cavernous).

Pathophysiology of BCVI

Different mechanisms of carotid and VAI contribute to a varied appearance on imaging. Blunt cerebrovascular dissection usually begins with a trauma-induced intimal tear or primary intramural hematoma.[27,28] With intimal injury, exposed subendothelial collagen initiates platelet aggregation to form thrombus (**Figs. 8** and **9**), which may produce vessel stenosis or occlusion or result in distal embolization (see **Fig. 8**). A dissecting hematoma within the media may propagate cranially to narrow or occlude the vessel (**Figs. 10** and **11**), or focally expand the adventitia to form a traumatic dissecting aneurysm (also referred to as "pseudoaneurysm").

IMAGING
Imaging Findings of BCVI

It is important to be familiar with the spectrum of findings and imaging pitfalls associated with the diagnosis of vascular injury on CTA, magnetic resonance (MR) imaging, MRA, and conventional angiography. Ultrasound imaging plays a limited role in diagnosis of cerebrovascular injury (see

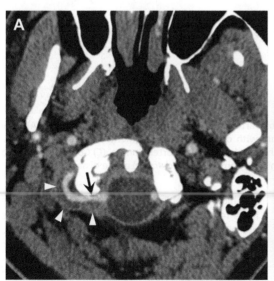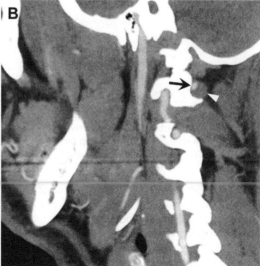

Fig. 4. Traumatic right vertebral dissection and intramural hematoma. (*A*) Axial and (*B*) sagittal CTA images show mild compression of the true lumen of the V3 segment of the right vertebral artery (*arrows*) by an extensive intramural hematoma (*arrowheads*). (*Courtesy of* Rihan Khan, MD.)

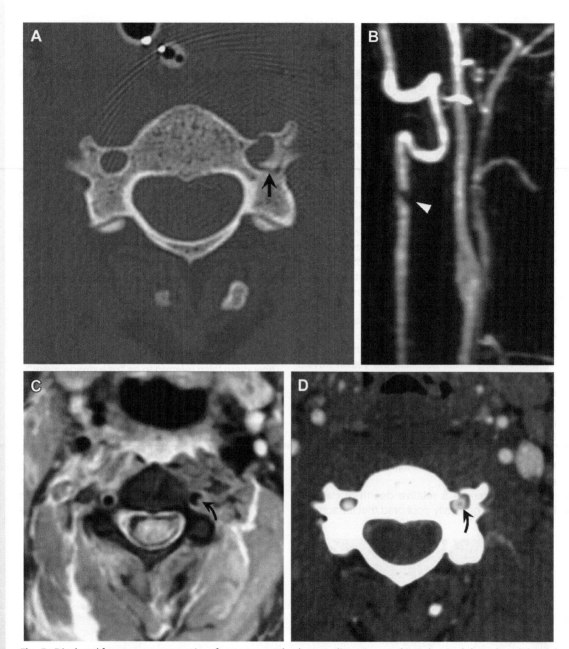

Fig. 5. Displaced foramen transversarium fracture, vertebral artery dissection, and intraluminal thrombus. (*A*) Axial CT shows a comminuted foramen transversarium fracture with displaced bone fragments (*arrow*). (*B*) Contrast-enhanced MRA reveals a dissection flap (*arrowhead*) within the left vertebral artery lumen. (*C*) Contrast-enhanced MR and (*D*) CTA images confirm the presence of intraluminal thrombus (*curved arrow*) at the dissection site.

Fig. 8), because of its poor detection of specific signs of BCVI lesions in the depth of the neck, where many ICA and VAI occur.[29]

In those patients at risk for BCVI, imaging of the entire cerebrovascular system should be performed from the aortic arch through the circle of Willis, as vessel injury may be remote from other signs of trauma. Another important imaging principle in the assessment for BCVI is to be aware of the high rate of multiple lesions. Several series have reported that up to 22% to 43% of injuries are bilateral (**Figs. 12** and **13**).[12,30–32]

Digital subtraction angiography (DSA) has been considered the gold standard for diagnostic evaluation of BCVI for many years (see **Figs. 2** and **13**). It is limited, however, by an inability to characterize the thickness and configuration of the arterial wall, the requirement to transport the patient

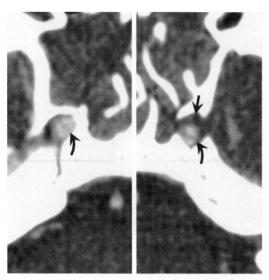

Fig. 6. Subtle bilateral ICA dissections with intimal flaps. The CTA image reveals bilateral ICA dissections with subtle intraluminal intimal flaps (*curved arrows*) consistent with a Denver grade 2 injury. Additionally seen is extraluminal hematoma (*arrow*) that does not compress the arterial lumen.

outside the emergency department, its invasive nature, and risk of procedural complications. The classic angiographic finding of dissection is an eccentric, long segment, tapered stenosis ("string sign") often associated with intimal irregularity (see Fig. 13). Focal narrowing with a more distal site of dilatation ("string-and-pearl sign") (see Fig. 13) can also be present.[33] Tapered stenosis with a concomitant dissecting aneurysm, occlusion, and isolated dissecting aneurysm are the most common imaging findings, in that order.[33] Pathognomonic imaging signs on DSA, such as intimal flap or a double lumen, are seen less commonly.

CTA provides the advantage of both high-spatial and high-contrast resolution of the arterial wall and lumen (see Figs. 2–9). In contradistinction to the 2 projections typically obtained with conventional angiography, CTA allows profiling of the entire 360° circumference of the arterial lumen, increasing sensitivity for detection of minor vessel injury. Inclusion of an unenhanced head CT is an essential component of a CTA protocol, to evaluate for associated intracranial hemorrhage and/or ischemia. These nonenhanced images may occasionally demonstrate injuries of the distal segments of injured carotid and vertebral arteries. Dissecting intramural hematomas can manifest on unenhanced CT as a hyperdense crescent-shaped mural lesion, often visualized near the skull base. On CTA, the same pathologic abnormality will be seen as luminal narrowing caused by crescentic intramural hematoma, which is usually

isodense to muscle.[34] Because this may be difficult to distinguish from atherosclerotic disease, recognizing that dissection will typically spare the carotid bulb is essential to making the correct diagnosis. Often the intramural hematoma causes overall enlargement of the external vessel diameter, despite narrowing of the lumen (see Figs. 2 and 3).[35] Other reliable signs of dissection on CTA include the identification of an intimal flap or dissecting aneurysm (see Figs. 2, 6, and 9). Multiplanar 2-dimensional (2D), curved planar 2D, and 3-dimensional (3D) reformations can be obtained to create images that are comparable to those seen with conventional angiography. Although these reformations are complementary, it is absolutely essential to evaluate the thin-section axial CT source images systematically for signs of vascular injury, as it may be obscured on 2D reconstructed images.

The MR imaging appearance of dissection is highly dependent on the age of the intramural hematoma, the surrounding tissues, and MR imaging sequences used for evaluation.[36] The MR imaging appearance of the hematoma will follow the known age-dependent signal intensity of paramagnetic iron (see Figs. 1, 3, 10, and 11). The intramural hematoma is usually most apparent in the subacute stage.[36,37] Subacute hematomas (containing methemoglobin) demonstrate characteristic findings on fat-suppressed T1-weighted images (see Fig. 10). The intramural hematoma will be seen as a high-intensity crescentic lesion adjacent to an eccentric flow void, which represents the residual lumen. The subacute intramural hematoma, with its short T1 values, will also be evident on noncontrast time-of-flight (TOF) MRA and can be mistaken for flow on these images (see Fig. 10). Phase-contrast and contrast-enhanced MRA will more clearly differentiate flow from the adjacent intramural hematoma. The intramural hematoma often causes overall enlargement of the external vessel diameter (see Figs. 3 and 10). Important pitfalls of MR imaging include the relative isointense appearance of acute (<7 days) and chronic (>2 months) hematoma on T1-weighted imaging, which blends in with surrounding tissues with fat suppression.[38] Dephasing and signal dropout on TOF images caused by turbulent flow in the horizontal petrous segment of the ICA can mimic intraluminal thrombus or dissection. Signal loss from in-plane flow or slab artifact on TOF imaging can also result in poor signal in horizontal segments of carotid or vertebral artery branches. Systematic evaluation of source images on TOF or contrast-enhanced MRA images is essential, to avoid missing subtle injury that may not be as apparent on reformations.

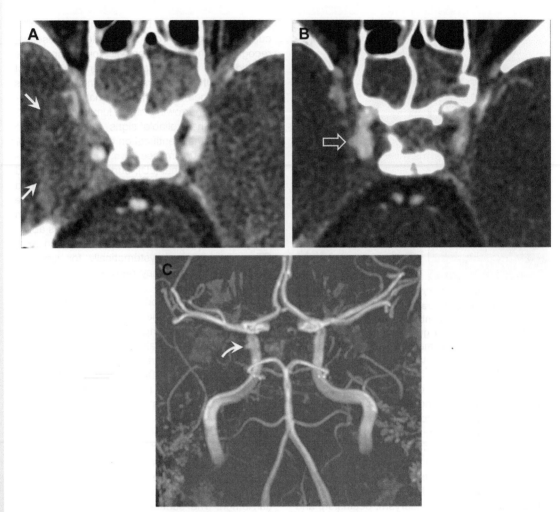

Fig. 7. Small traumatic internal carotid pseudoaneurysm. (*A, B*) CTA images reveal a large parasellar epidural hematoma (*arrows*) with a probable small traumatic ICA pseudoaneurysm (*open arrow*). (*C*) The aneurysm (*curved arrow*) is confirmed on a 3D-TOF MIP image. Extensive central skull base fractures likely partially avulsed an intracavernous ICA branch from the parent artery.

Color Duplex ultrasound has a limited role in the evaluation of BCVI patients, as 90% of traumatic lesions occur in acoustically nonassessable segments of the carotid and vertebral arteries.[29] The cephalad parts of the extracranial ICA and VA are difficult to image, requiring use of low-frequency sector transducers and reliance mainly on hemodynamic abnormalities for diagnosis of dissection. Most dissecting aneurysms are missed.[39] That said, specific signs of dissection may be detected in the more accessible proximal ICA, with mural hematoma manifesting as a thickened hypoechoic vessel wall on B-mode or high-frequency sector transducers.[40] Intimal flaps and double lumens are occasionally depicted (see **Fig. 8**).

BCVI Classification

Traumatic cerebrovascular injuries can be classified by the location of injury (intracranial vs extracranial) and/or the extent of vessel wall involvement. The mildest form of injury is merely extrinsic compression of the lumen by extramural hematoma, (**Fig. 14**) without a true tear of the vessel wall. True vascular tears may affect just the intima, both the intima and the media, or may extend through the entire thickness of the vessel wall. The greater the extent of wall disruption, the more abnormal the vessel configuration will appear on imaging studies (**Figs. 15–20**).

The emerging literature on blunt BCVI in the early to mid-1990s prompted the call for a formal injury grading scale that could stratify injuries

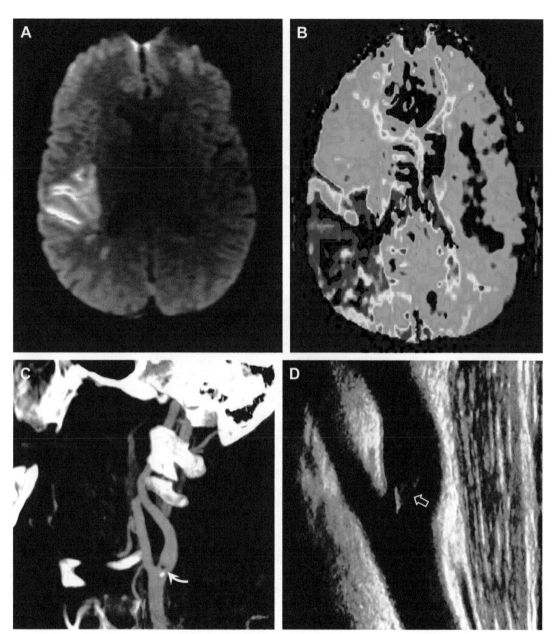

Fig. 8. Subtle traumatic dissection with intraluminal thrombus and embolic stroke. (*A*) Diffusion-weighted and (*B*) perfusion MR images. This patient presented with a right hemispheric infarct 24 hours following a motor vehicle accident and blunt anterior neck trauma. Note the size of the perfusion deficit is greater than the size of the diffusion-weighted image abnormality, indicating an ischemic penumbra. (*C*) Sagittal 2D reformatted CTA image reveals a filling defect due to thrombus (*curved arrow*) within the lumen of the ICA without other abnormality. (*D*) Duplex sonogram confirms the presence of intraluminal clot (*open arrow*) likely due to a subtle traumatic dissection.

by type, location, and neurologic presentation, as well as provide prognostic and therapeutic value.[2] As a result, a cerebrovascular injury grading scale was developed at Denver Health Medical Center in 1999, based on the conventional arteriographic imaging appearance of lesions. This Denver grading scale has been widely used in subsequent large prospective and retrospective series throughout the surgical and trauma literature. This literature has demonstrated that different injury grades may have differing risks of morbidity and mortality, distinct responses to therapy, and differing final neurologic outcomes.[9,11,12,29,32,41–44]

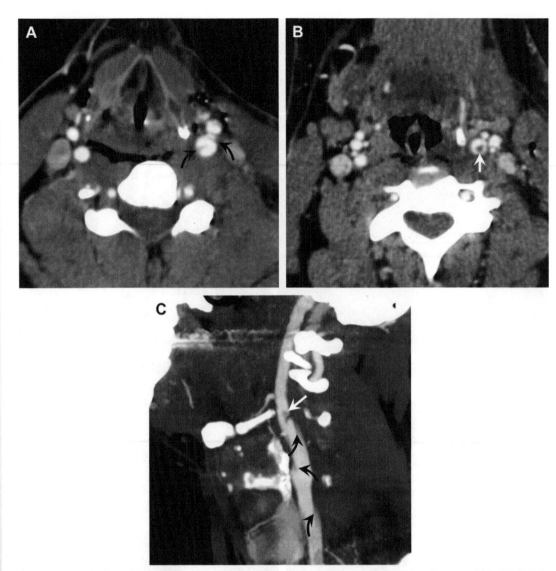

Fig. 9. Traumatic dissection with intraluminal thrombus. Axial (*A, B*) and sagittal 2D reformatted (*C*) CTA images reveal a complex dissection of the proximal ICA (*black curved arrows*) with evidence of intraluminal thrombus (*arrow*), indicating a Denver grade 2 injury. This patient is at great risk for subsequent distal embolization unless treated with antithrombotic agents.

Broadly, the Denver grading scale (**Table 1**) categorizes lesions as nonhemodynamically significant injuries (grade I) (see **Fig. 12**), potentially hemodynamically significant dissections and hematomas (grade II) (see **Figs. 5, 6, 8–13**), pseudoaneurysms (grade III) (see **Figs. 2, 3, 7, and 18**), occlusions (grade IV) (see **Figs. 1 and 20**), and vessel transections with free extravasation (grade V) (see **Figs. 15–17** and **19**). Specifically, grade I injury is defined as irregularity of the vessel wall or a dissection with less than 25% luminal stenosis. Grade 2 injuries consist of a dissection of the vessel wall with greater than 25% luminal

stenosis or a dissection with a visible intimal flap.[30] Some have proposed grade V injuries be separated into noncontained rupture with free extravasation and intravascular rupture (arteriovenous fistula).[45]

Role of Imaging in BCVI Screening

A significant percentage of BCVI patients may present with an initially asymptomatic period.[1,7,12,13] Thus, a window of opportunity exists to treat traumatic lesions before irreversible, catastrophic complications develop (see **Fig. 20**). Identifying

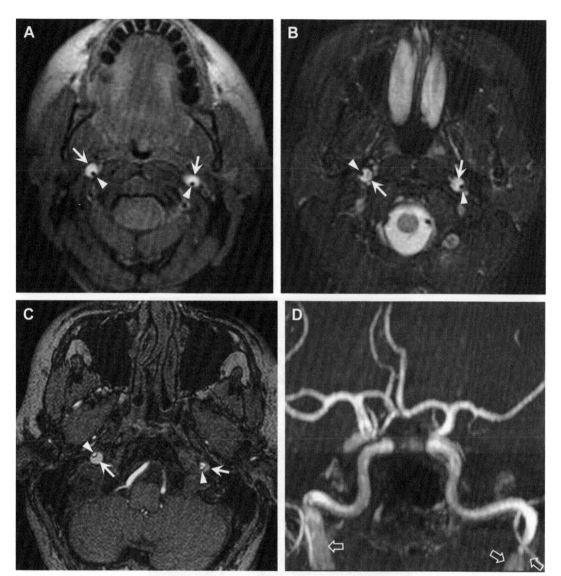

Fig. 10. Bilateral ICA dissections causing severe luminal compromise. Axial proton density-weighted (PD-W) (*A*) and T2-weighted (*B*) MR images as well as source (*C*) and MIP (*D*) images from a 3D-TOF MRA demonstrate bilateral ICA dissections 1 week following neck trauma. Note that the true lumens (*arrowheads*) are severely narrowed by intramural hematoma (*arrows*). The intramural hematoma is hyperintense and very visible on the PD-W and T2-weighted images. The hematoma is also hyperintense on the T1-weighted source image, which can be mistaken for flow on the MIP image (*open arrows*).

BCVI before the onset of symptoms is the primary goal of imaging, to facilitate prompt initiation of adequate antithrombotic medical therapy. Early effective treatment has been demonstrated to improve neurologic outcomes and prevent stroke.[1,7,12,13] Diagnosis and implementation of treatment during this silent period has been the "holy grail" of BCVI, driving the use of aggressive and liberal screening protocols to capture this population. Although challenges and controversy exist in defining the population at risk, the integral

role of noninvasive high-resolution CT screening in both asymptomatic and symptomatic patients has been clearly established.

Several prior studies have looked at various clinical and radiographic criteria to try and predict which patients with craniocervical trauma are at a high risk of cerebrovascular injury. The 2 most widely implemented screening protocols are based on the Memphis criteria, developed by Miller and colleagues,[10] and the Denver criteria, developed by Biffl and colleagues.[7,30] Most

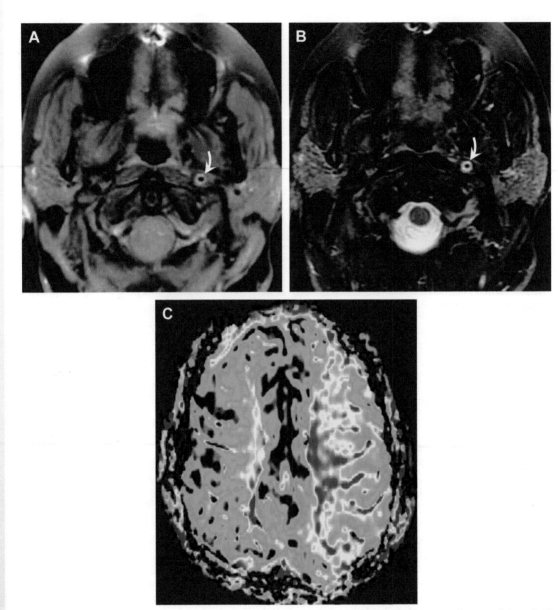

Fig. 11. Left ICA dissection with severe luminal compromise and perfusion deficit. Axial PD-W (*A*) and T2-weighted (*B*) MR images as well as a perfusion MR image (*C*) demonstrate a left ICA dissection with circumferential intramural thrombus (*curved arrows*). The carotid lumen is severely narrowed and there is prolonged transit time on the perfusion image, indicating a risk for subsequent infarct.

recently, the Eastern and Western Trauma Associations have published recommended screening algorithms based on systematic analysis, observational studies, and expert opinion.[29,41] Despite evidence for improved BCVI detection with aggressive screening algorithms, retrospective studies have demonstrated that up to 20% to 34% of BCVI patients still fail to meet established screening criteria.[7,23,30,46] This high percentage of potentially "missed" diagnoses indicates significant room for improvement of existing algorithms.

Craniofacial fractures have been repeatedly implicated as a cause of BCVI in numerous retrospective studies, particularly CAI, although the association has been poorly characterized.[1,2,12,46,47] The Western and Eastern Trauma Associations currently recommend screening all patients with cervical spine, basilar skull, and Le Fort II or III facial fractures for the presence of BCVI. This recommendation, however, was based on retrospective series, which established facial fracture diagnoses from review of International Classification of Diseases, Ninth Revision (ICD-9) codes,

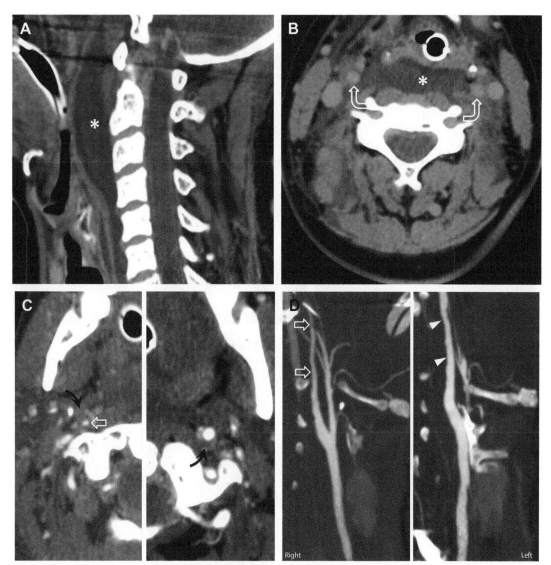

Fig. 12. Bilateral ICA dissections with "string" signs. Sagittal (*A*) and axial (*B*) CT images demonstrate a large retropharyngeal hematoma (*asterisk*), which extends laterally to the carotid spaces (*curved open arrows*), suggesting the possibility of traumatic BCVI and the need for a CTA. (*C*) Axial and (*D*) bilateral sagittal CTA images reveal intramural hematoma (*curved arrows*) causing severe right (Denver grade 2) (*open arrows*) and mild left (Denver grade 1) (*arrowheads*) luminal compromise (string sign).

rather than evaluation and classification of facial fractures by retrospective review of available clinical imaging.

Several small studies have attempted to address the association between facial fractures and BCAI but have lacked the power to perform statistical analysis.[48–50] A recent large retrospective series of 4398 patients with blunt mechanism facial fractures attempted to determine whether specific patterns of facial fracture are associated with an increased risk of carotid artery injury, and if so, whether they could be a valuable contribution to the screening criteria in place.[44] Results indicated that bilateral fractures of any "facial third," complex midface fractures including all Le Fort type injuries, and subcondylar mandibular fractures (especially in the setting of associated skull base fracture) conferred an increased risk of BCAI (see **Figs. 4, 6,** and **12**).[44] Analysis of adding Le Fort type I injury to existing screening criteria demonstrated resultant increased sensitivity, although positive and negative predictive values remained unchanged.

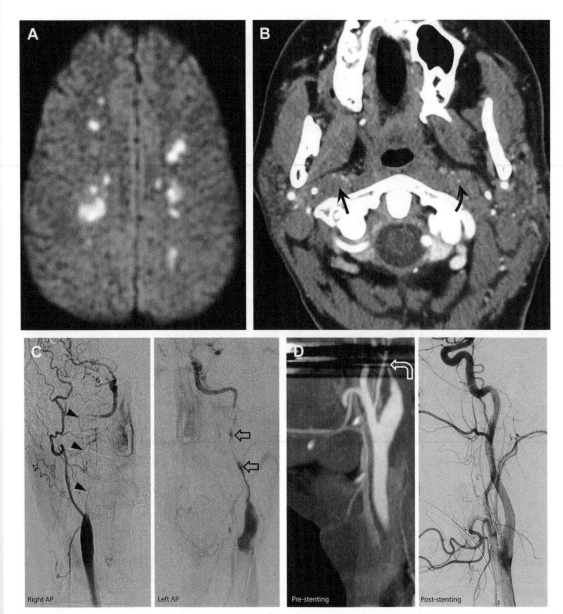

Fig. 13. Bilateral terminal zone infarcts due to ICA dissections with "string" signs. (*A*) Axial diffusion-weighted image demonstrates bilateral acute terminal zone infarcts compatible with hypoperfusion, raising the strong possibility of bilateral ICA injury. (*B*) Axial CTA image confirms a left carotid string sign (*curved arrow*) and possible right carotid occlusion (*arrow*). (*C*) Bilateral carotid angiograms demonstrate severe bilateral tapered ICA stenoses (Denver grade 2) due to ICA dissections. There is severe right ICA luminal compromise (string sign) (*arrowheads*) and an irregular left ICA stenosis with several focal dilatations (string-and-pearl sign) (*open arrows*). (*D*) Prestenting and poststenting images of the left ICA reveal marked improvement of the severe left ICA stenosis (*curved open arrow*).

A retrospective series of 1882 patients with craniocervical trauma similarly evaluated patterns of craniofacial fracture and association with BCVI, using relative risk (RR) calculations.[45] Mandible and midface fractures, when considered as a whole, only mildly increased the risk for BCVI (RR 1.4% and 1.3%, respectively). However, when subsets of midface fractures were considered, a markedly elevated risk was demonstrated for fractures of the sphenotemporal buttress (RR 3.9%) and orbital roof/rim fractures that extended into the central skull base (RR 2.8%). Interestingly,

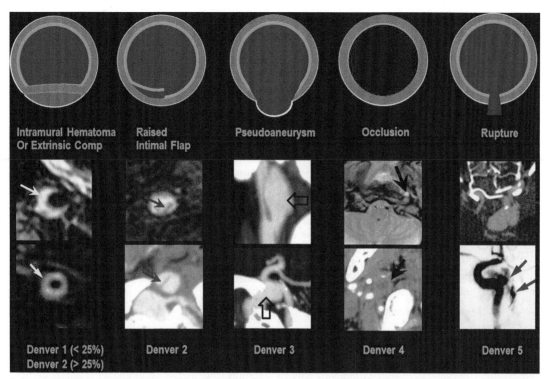

Fig. 14. Pathologic abnormality and classification of traumatic cerebrovascular injury. This diagram demonstrates the most common types of traumatic vascular injuries, their Denver grade, and their appearances on CTA, MRA, and angiogram images. Denver grade 1 is characterized by less than 25% luminal compromise by intramural or extramural hematoma. Grade 2 indicates either greater than 25% luminal compromise (*yellow arrows*) or a raised intimal flap (*red arrows*). Denver grade 3 is due to a pseudoaneurysm (*open arrows*), whereas grade 4 indicates a vessel occlusion (*blue arrows*). Free rupture and extravasation is a grade 5 injury (*red arrows*).

Le Fort fractures by themselves did not correlate with significantly higher risk unless they were associated with fractures of the carotid canal. Facial or skull base fractures of any type extending into the carotid canal, especially when associated with greater than 2-mm displacement, were associated with a much higher risk of BCVI (RR 5.2%). Of note, atlanto-occipital subluxation/dislocation conferred the highest risk, wherein 1 in 5 patients had vertebral artery dissection, pseudoaneurysm, vessel transection, or arteriovenous fistula.

Thus, emerging data suggest it is possible to stratify patients into higher BCVI risk categories by evaluating them with initial high-resolution head, maxillofacial, and cervical spine CT examinations, although further work in uncovering mechanistic relations between craniofacial injury patterns and BCAI is needed to maximize diagnostic yield and better guide prompt management.

Role of Imaging in BCVI Diagnosis

Imaging not only plays a vital role in identification of patients at high risk for BCVI that require further vascular workup but also in characterizing the injury itself (**Box 1, Tables 2** and **3**). Among other remaining key and somewhat controversial issues, debate continues in regards to the optimal diagnostic modality.

As discussed, conventional angiography is the gold standard for detecting vascular injury. Liberalized use of 4-vessel DSA has raised concerns, however, due to its invasive, time-consuming, and resource-intensive nature.[7,13,31,32,46] The risks of invasive DSA are not inconsequential, with the accepted complication rate (including stroke) ranging between 0.1% and 1.0% of angiographic studies performed to detect BCVI.[13,31]

In contrast to DSA, CTA can be performed in many hospitals without the necessity of transporting the patient outside the emergency department. With the dissemination of more advanced multidetector CT (MDCT) scanners ($\geq$16 channels), CTA has emerged as the preferred diagnostic modality in most institutions.[51] Studies comparing 16-slice MDCT and conventional DSA have suffered from diagnostic inconsistencies, which in part appear related to the experience of the radiologists

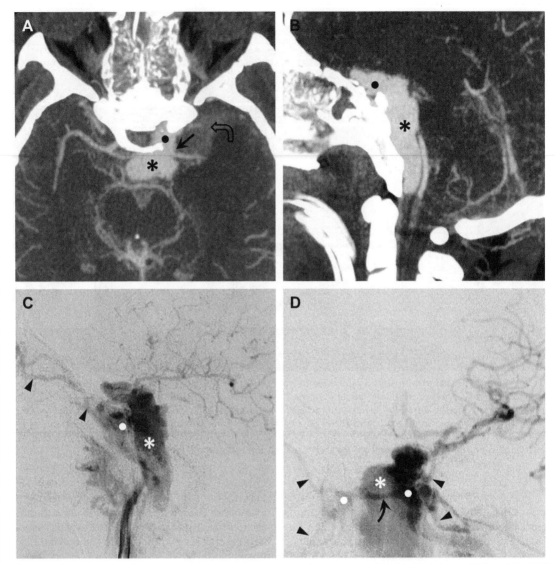

Fig. 15. ICA transection, free contrast extravasation, and carotid-cavernous fistula. (A) Axial and (B) sagittal MIP images from a CTA demonstrate extensive dilatation of the left cavernous sinus (•) as well as extravasation of contrast into a semi-contained prepontine hematoma (*asterisk*) and subarachnoid space (*curved open arrow*). The left ICA (*arrow*) is not well seen due to the ICA transection. (C) Lateral and (D) anteroposterior angiogram images confirm free extravasation of contrast into the prepontine cistern (•), early entry of contrast into the cavernous sinuses (*asterisk*), and filling of the superior and inferior ophthalmic veins (*arrowheads*). Note that contrast fills both of the cavernous sinuses via an anterior intercavernous vein (*curved arrow*).

interpreting the traumatic BCVI studies. Some investigators reported CTA sensitivities and specificity in detecting BCVI of up to 100%, although one study reported sensitivity of 64-slice MDCT at just 54%.[52–54] In contradistinction, Fakhry and colleagues[55] reported oversensitivity (high false positive rate) of CTA. Although CTA may be slightly less accurate than conventional angiography in detecting subtle intimal injuries, it provides rapid and accurate assessment of vascular injuries and is considered the study of choice for asymptomatic patients deemed at high risk of vascular injury. In patients with normal or equivocal findings on CTA, angiography may be warranted to definitively exclude an injury when clinical suspicion is high. More recently, whole-body MDCT protocols have been proposed to evaluate both vascular injury and cervical spine integrity with one spiral

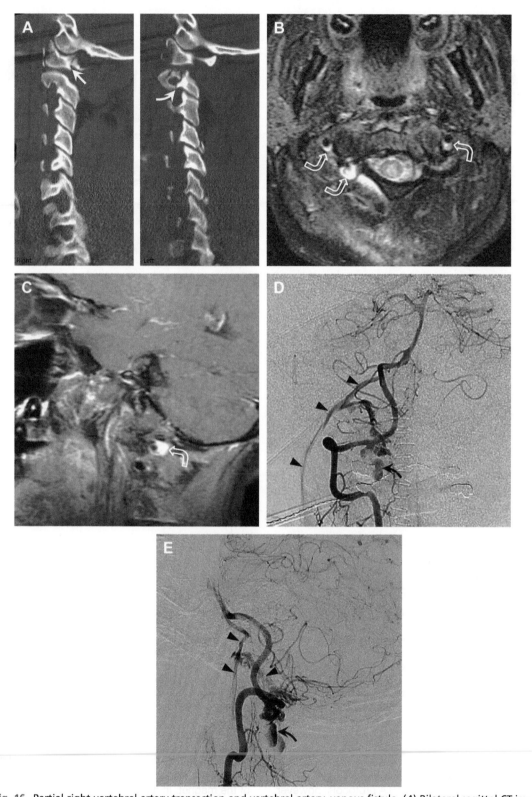

Fig. 16. Partial right vertebral artery transection and vertebral artery–venous fistula. (*A*) Bilateral sagittal CT images demonstrate fractures of the right C1 posterior arch (*white arrow*) and left C2 foramen transversarium (*curved white arrow*), both of which are known high-risk radiographic findings for BCVI. Axial (*B*) and right sagittal (*C*) T1-weighted fat-suppressed contrast-enhanced MR images reveal areas of intramural contrast extravasation (*curved white arrows*) at sites of vascular injury. Lateral (*D*) and anteroposterior (*E*) angiogram images reveal early entry of contrast into the perimedullary venous plexus (*arrowheads*), confirming an arteriovenous fistula. Additionally present are free contrast extravasation and loculated collections of contrast (*curved arrow*) within the paravertebral soft tissues, representing a Denver grade 5 injury.

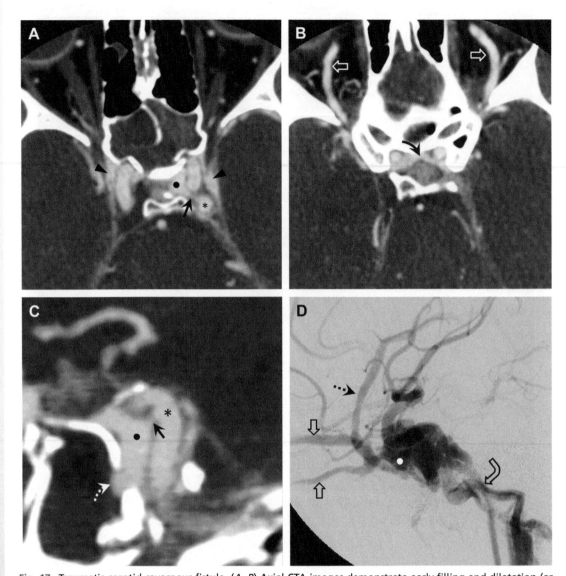

Fig. 17. Traumatic carotid-cavernous fistula. (*A, B*) Axial CTA images demonstrate early filling and dilatation (arterialization) of the cavernous sinuses (*arrowhead*) due to fistulous connection (*arrow*) between the left ICA (*asterisk*) and a large cavernous sinus venous varix (•). There is dilatation of the superior ophthalmic veins (*open arrows*). Bilateral cavernous sinus involvement is due to a large patent anterior intercavernous vein (*curved arrow*). (*C*) Sagittal 2D reconstructed CTA image confirms the fistulous connection (*arrow*) between the ICA (*asterisk*) and venous varix (•). The patient is at very high risk of future epistaxis due to extension of the venous varix through a fracture into the sphenoid sinus (*curved dashed arrow*). (*D*) Lateral angiogram confirms early entry of contrast into the cavernous sinus (•), ophthalmic veins (*open arrows*), sphenoparietal sinus (*dashed arrow*), and inferior petrosal sinus (*curved open arrow*).

acquisition and contrast dose.[56] The diagnostic quality of this technique has not yet been proven comparable to individual CTA protocols, however.

MRA with MR imaging is a capable alternative to CTA, with both relative advantages and disadvantages. Disadvantages of MRA include the requirement of patient transportation outside the emergency department, a somewhat time-consuming screening process of the patient for

contraindications to the magnet, and greater difficulty of monitoring injured patients inside the bore of the magnet. In addition, MRA may not be available in some centers; high-quality images are more difficult to obtain, and the interpretation of the study requires more experience. At least one prospective study demonstrated MR imaging in combination with MRA to have excellent sensitivity and specificity in detecting carotid artery

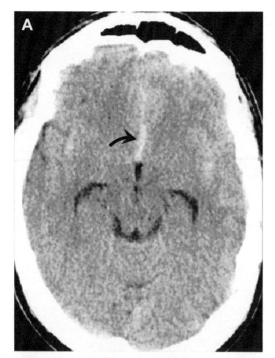

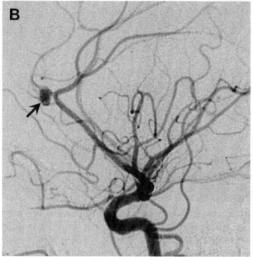

Fig. 18. Traumatic pericallosal aneurysm. (A) Axial CT images demonstrate extensive posttraumatic subarachnoid hemorrhage within the anterior interhemispheric fissure (*curved arrow*), greater than expected considering the degree of the patients' other intracranial injuries. A high index of suspicion for traumatic CVI is indicated and additional workup is needed. (B) Lateral angiogram depicts a traumatic pericallosal aneurysm (*arrow*). Posttraumatic aneurysms in this location likely result from partial avulsion of cortical arterial branches from the pericallosal artery due to excessive shift of the frontal lobes in relation to the more fixed corpus callosum.

dissection (95% and 99%, respectively) (see **Figs. 3, 5, 10,** and **12**) compared with conventional DSA, although it fared poorly with VAI detection (sensitivity and specificity of 60% and 58%, respectively).[57] Numerous other studies report less favorable MR imaging/MRA results.[23,31,57] MRA has not gained general acceptance as the preferred screening modality, but may be the study of choice for the evaluation of BCVI patients with symptoms suggestive of trauma-induced stroke (see **Fig. 1**). MR imaging and MRA are especially useful for vascular injuries causing ischemic complications, identifying coexisting infarcts, and evaluating for perfusion defects (see **Figs. 1, 3, 8,** and **11**).

Duplex ultrasonography has a limited role in the assessment of cerebrovascular injuries because of its limitations in visualizing the entire cerebrovascular system, its inability to characterize direct signs of injury in most cases, and poor overall sensitivity and specificity. Consequently, ultrasound is not recommended as a screening tool for possible BCVI.

BCVI Treatment and Follow-Up

The development of the Denver grading scale enabled investigation into prognostic and treatment implications associated with the varying degrees of traumatic cerebrovascular injury.[30] The primary management strategies for BCVI have included observation, surgical repair, antithrombotic drugs, and endovascular therapy. Although consensus on optimal patient treatment and follow-up is lacking, decisions and recommendations typically take into consideration patient symptoms and injury location/grade (anatomic description).

BCVI has been historically associated with high morbidities and mortalities when untreated. Management through observation alone is therefore not recommended, unless there are significant comorbidities contraindicating more aggressive treatment strategies.

Given the pathophysiology of intimal injury and subsequent platelet aggregation in BCVI, it is not surprising that antithrombotic agents have been used in an attempt to improve patient outcomes. Although the literature reveals some contradictory results, the overall body of evidence has indicated that the use of antithrombotic agents in BCVI can significantly improve mortality and prevent permanent neurologic deficits in patients.[1,13,32] No direct, controlled comparison studies of heparin versus antiplatelet agents have been performed to demonstrate superiority in outcome, although one of several subgroup analyses showed slight

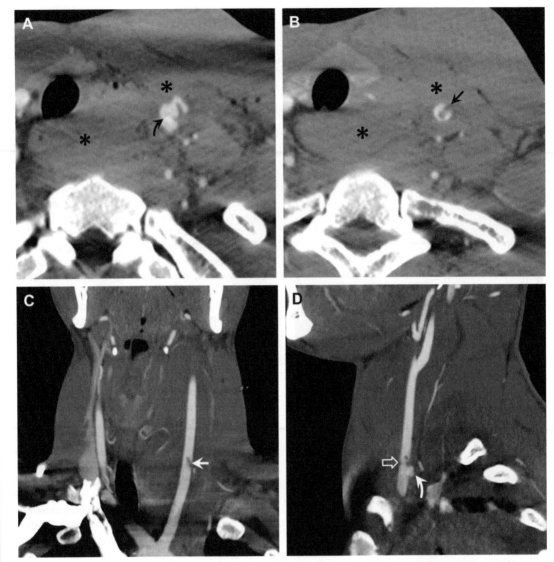

Fig. 19. Incomplete left common carotid artery transection. (*A*, *B*) Axial CTA images demonstrate extensive retrotracheal and carotid space hematoma (*asterisks*) with traumatic disruption of the left common carotid artery and a large pseudoaneurysm (*curved black arrow*). A large intraluminal dissection flap (*black arrow*) is also present. (*C*) Coronal and (*D*) sagittal 2D reconstructed CTA images confirm near complete vessel transection (*open arrow*), pseudoaneurysm formation (*curved white arrow*), and a large intimal flap (*white arrow*).

improvement in BCVI neurologic outcome with heparin treatment.[7] Recent Eastern Association for the Surgery of Trauma management guidelines advocate treatment of grade 1 and grade 2 injuries with either heparin or antiplatelet therapy, citing equivalent efficacy.[29] Anticoagulation is not without risk. Serious bleeding complications have been reported, particularly in patients with documented intracranial hemorrhage before initiation of therapy.[7] Conservative anticoagulation protocols have been recommended, although no

optimal regimen or duration of therapy has been established.[23,29]

Interestingly, evidence suggests it is the lower grade lesions (Denver grading scale I and II) that are the most dynamic, with 8% of grade I and 43% of grade II BCVI lesions progressing on follow-up DSA imaging in the 7 to 10 days following the injury.[31] Approximately 60% of patients with grade I and II injuries required change in management. These findings give credence to routine follow-up of such lesions, either by

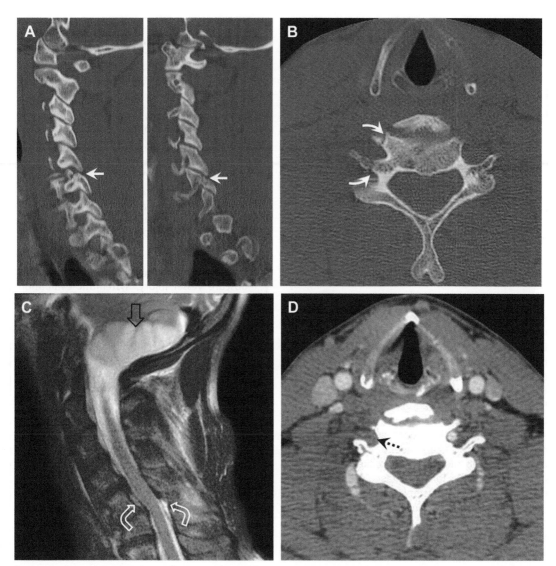

Fig. 20. Right vertebral artery occlusion and "asymptomatic" posterior inferior cerebellar artery infarct. Sagittal (A) and axial (B) CT images of a chiropractor who sustained a motor vehicle accident demonstrate fractures (arrows) of the right superior articular facet and lateral mass of C5. There is involvement of the C5 foramen transversarium (curved arrows). There is no subluxation on the sagittal images. (C) A sagittal T2-weighted MR imaging scan was obtained to rule out ligamentous injury. There is new C5–C6 vertebral subluxation and evidence of ligamentous injury (curved open arrows). An "asymptomatic" posterior inferior cerebellar artery infarct (open arrow) is present. (D) Axial CTA image confirms occlusion of the right vertebral artery (dashed arrow).

conventional DSA or by noninvasive (CTA, MR/MRA) imaging.

Complete vessel occlusions (grade IV lesions) may recanalize as part of their natural history, although they do not typically do so in the early postinjury period. Despite a high risk of stroke in complete vessel occlusion, anticoagulation has been demonstrated to improve outcomes in this population.[30] The optimal agent, duration, and end point in therapy have not been established for this group.

Grade III lesions (dissecting aneurysm) place the patient at risk for a thromboembolic event and progression to vessel occlusion or rupture. Carrying the highest rate of mortality, grade V lesions are devastating and intervention is often preempted by patient demise (see **Fig. 15**).[30] These higher grade lesions have been found to rarely heal with

Table 1	
BCVI Denver grading scale	
Injury Grade	**Description**
I	Luminal irregularity or dissection with <25% luminal narrowing
II	Dissection or intramural hematoma with ≥25% luminal narrowing, intraluminal thrombus, or raised intimal flap
III	Pseudoaneurysm
IV	Occlusion
V	Transection with free extravasation

From Biffl WL, Moore EE, Offner PJ, et al. Blunt carotid arterial injuries: implications of a new grading scale. J Trauma 1999;47(5):845–53; with permission.

antithrombotic therapy alone; therefore, surgical management has been traditionally advocated. In the last decade, however, endovascular therapy has been used much more frequently, because of the number of BCVIs that are not amenable to open surgical treatment.[11] DiCocco and colleagues[11] advocate aggressive endovascular therapy for grade II, III, and V lesions, citing after-diagnosis stroke rates similar to that of medical therapy (4%), despite treating lesions associated with much higher stroke risks. Clear risk-benefit ratios for endovascular treatments have not been well established, and concerns have been raised regarding stent-related complications and the need for expensive dual antiplatelet therapy following placement of drug-eluting stents.[58]

Box 1
BCVI imaging pearls and pitfalls

Pearls

- There is a high rate of BCVI multifocality (up to 43%).
- CTA has emerged as the preferred diagnostic modality for BCVI in most institutions.
- Vessel injury may be remote from other signs of trauma; thus, imaging from the aortic arch through the circle of Willis is essential.
- Mural hematoma may mimic the appearance of atherosclerotic plaque on CTA; however, in contradistinction to atherosclerotic disease, BCVI will typically spare the carotid bulb.

Pitfalls

- Multiplanar 2D and 3D reformations may obscure vessel injury; systematic evaluation of thin-section axial CT and MR imaging source images for signs of vascular injury is crucial.
- On noncontrast TOF MRA, BCVI manifested as subacute intramural hematoma (with its short T1 values) can be mistaken for flow. Phase contrast and contrast-enhanced MRA will more clearly differentiate flow from the adjacent intramural hematoma.
- On fat-suppressed T1-weighted MR imaging, the relative isointense appearance of acute (<7 days) and chronic (>2 months) hematoma blends in with surrounding tissues, making it difficult to detect.
- Dephasing and signal dropout on TOF MRA images caused by turbulent flow in the horizontal petrous segment of the ICA can mimic intraluminal thrombus or dissection.

Table 2		
Imaging screening criteria for BCVI (asymptomatic patients)		
Screening Criteria Adapted from Biffl et al[41]	**Denver Modification of Screening Criteria[41]**	**Memphis Screening Criteria[10]**
• Displaced midface or complex mandibular fracture (in setting of cervical rotation/hyperflexion or extension) • Cervical vertebral body fracture • Basilar skull fracture involving the carotid canal • Fracture in proximity to ICA or VA • Diffuse axonal injury • Anoxic brain Injury	• Displaced Le Fort II or III fracture • Cervical spine fracture with: ○ Subluxation ○ Extension into transverse foramen ○ C1–C3 involvement • Basilar skull fracture with carotid canal extension • Diffuse axonal injury • Anoxic brain injury	• Le Fort II or III fracture • Cervical spine fracture • Skull base fracture involving the foramen lacerum

Table 3
Craniofacial trauma radiologic risk factors for BCVI

Mundinger et al[44]	Alsheik et al[45]
• Bilateral fractures of any "facial third" • Complex midface fracture (Le Fort I, II, III) • Subcondylar mandibular fracture (in the setting of associated skull base fracture)	• Sphenotemporal buttress fracture • Orbital roof/rim fracture with central skull base extension • Facial or skull base fractures with carotid canal extension (especially with >2 mm displacement) • Atlanto-occipital subluxation/dislocation (1 in 5 patients had VA injury)

SUMMARY

Significant recent progress has been made in the recognition, screening, diagnosis, and treatment of BCVI. Although controversy still exists as to optimal screening algorithms and best diagnostic modality, the vital and growing role of noninvasive imaging in identifying patients at high risk for BCVI and in characterizing the injury itself has been clearly established. There has been promising early work in stratifying BCVI patients into risk categories by initially evaluating them with high-resolution head, maxillofacial, and cervical CT examinations with the ultimate goal of maximizing diagnostic yield and enabling prompt initiation of therapy. Further work is needed, however, to delineate the mechanistic relationship between craniofacial fractures and BCVI.

REFERENCES

1. Fabian TC, Patton JH Jr, Croce MA, et al. Blunt carotid injury. Importance of early diagnosis and anticoagulant therapy. Ann Surg 1996;223(5):513–22 [discussion: 522–5].

2. Cogbill TH, Moore EE, Meissner M, et al. The spectrum of blunt injury to the carotid artery: a multi-center perspective. J Trauma 1994;37(3):473–9.

3. Davis JW, Holbrook TL, Hoyt DB, et al. Blunt carotid artery dissection: incidence, associated injuries, screening, and treatment. J Trauma 1990;30(12):1514–7.

4. Martin RF, Eldrup-Jorgensen J, Clark DE, et al. Blunt trauma to the carotid arteries. J Vasc Surg 1991;14(6):789–93 [discussion: 793–5].

5. Ramadan F, Rutledge R, Oller D, et al. Carotid artery trauma: a review of contemporary trauma center experiences. J Vasc Surg 1995;21(1):46–55 [discussion: 55–6].

6. Mutze S, Rademacher G, Matthes G, et al. Blunt cerebrovascular injury in patients with blunt multiple trauma: diagnostic accuracy of duplex Doppler US and early CT angiography. Radiology 2005;237(3):884–92.

7. Biffl WL, Moore EE, Ryu RK, et al. The unrecognized epidemic of blunt carotid arterial injuries: early diagnosis improves neurologic outcome. Ann Surg 1998;228(4):462–70.

8. Berne JD, Norwood SH, McAuley CE, et al. The high morbidity of blunt cerebrovascular injury in an unscreened population: more evidence of the need for mandatory screening protocols. J Am Coll Surg 2001;192(3):314–21.

9. Emmett KP, Fabian TC, DiCocco JM, et al. Improving the screening criteria for blunt cerebrovascular injury: the appropriate role for computed tomography angiography. J Trauma 2011;70(5):1058–63 [discussion: 1063–5].

10. Miller PR, Fabian TC, Croce MA, et al. Prospective screening for blunt cerebrovascular injuries: analysis of diagnostic modalities and outcomes. Ann Surg 2002;236(3):386–93 [discussion: 393–5].

11. DiCocco JM, Fabian TC, Emmett KP, et al. Optimal outcomes for patients with blunt cerebrovascular injury (BCVI): tailoring treatment to the lesion. J Am Coll Surg 2011;212(4):549–57 [discussion: 557–9].

12. Biffl WL, Moore EE, Elliott JP, et al. The devastating potential of blunt vertebral arterial injuries. Ann Surg 2000;231(5):672–81.

13. Miller PR, Fabian TC, Bee TK, et al. Blunt cerebrovascular injuries: diagnosis and treatment. J Trauma 2001;51(2):279–85 [discussion: 285–6].

14. Crissey MM, Bernstein EF. Delayed presentation of carotid intimal tear following blunt craniocervical trauma. Surgery 1974;75(4):543–9.

15. Arthurs ZM, Starnes BW. Blunt carotid and vertebral artery injuries. Injury 2008;39(11):1232–41.

16. Cothren CC, Moore EE, Ray CE Jr, et al. Cervical spine fracture patterns mandating screening to rule out blunt cerebrovascular injury. Surgery 2007;141(1):76–82.

17. Anson J, Crowell RM. Cervicocranial arterial dissection. Neurosurgery 1991;29(1):89–96.

18. Zelenock GB, Kazmers A, Whitehouse WM Jr, et al. Extracranial internal carotid artery dissections: noniatrogenic traumatic lesions. Arch Surg 1982;117(4):425–32.

19. Moar JJ. Traumatic rupture of the cervical carotid arteries: an autopsy and histopathological study of 200 cases. Forensic Sci Int 1987;34(4):227–44.

20. Mulloy JP, Flick PA, Gold RE. Blunt carotid injury: a review. Radiology 1998;207(3):571–85.

21. Kang SY, Lin EM, Marentette LJ. Importance of complete pterygomaxillary separation in the le fort I osteotomy: an anatomic report. Skull Base 2009;19(4):273–7.

22. Arnold M, Bousser MG, Fahrni G, et al. Vertebral artery dissection: presenting findings and predictors of outcome. Stroke 2006;37(10):2499–503.

23. Biffl WL, Ray CE Jr, Moore EE, et al. Noninvasive diagnosis of blunt cerebrovascular injuries: a preliminary report. J Trauma 2002;53(5):850–6.

24. Parent AD, Harkey HL, Touchstone DA, et al. Lateral cervical spine dislocation and vertebral artery injury. Neurosurgery 1992;31(3):501–9.

25. Willis BK, Greiner F, Orrison WW, et al. The incidence of vertebral artery injury after midcervical spine fracture or subluxation. Neurosurgery 1994; 34(3):435–41 [discussion: 441–2].

26. McKevitt EC, Kirkpatrick AW, Vertesi L, et al. Identifying patients at risk for intracranial and extracranial blunt carotid injuries. Am J Surg 2002;183(5): 566–70.

27. Schievink WI, Piepgras DG, McCaffrey TV, et al. Surgical treatment of extracranial internal carotid artery dissecting aneurysms. Neurosurgery 1994; 35(5):809–15 [discussion: 815–6].

28. Muller BT, Luther B, Hort W, et al. Surgical treatment of 50 carotid dissections: indications and results. J Vasc Surg 2000;31(5):980–8.

29. Bromberg WJ, Collier BC, Diebel LN, et al. Blunt cerebrovascular injury practice management guidelines: the Eastern Association for the Surgery of Trauma. J Trauma 2010;68(2):471–7.

30. Biffl WL, Moore EE, Offner PJ, et al. Blunt carotid arterial injuries: implications of a new grading scale. J Trauma 1999;47(5):845–53.

31. Biffl WL, Ray CE Jr, Moore EE, et al. Treatment-related outcomes from blunt cerebrovascular injuries: importance of routine follow-up arteriography. Ann Surg 2002;235(5):699–706 [discussion: 706–7].

32. Cothren CC, Moore EE, Biffl WL, et al. Anticoagulation is the gold standard therapy for blunt carotid injuries to reduce stroke rate. Arch Surg 2004; 139(5):540–5 [discussion: 545–6].

33. Houser OW, Mokri B, Sundt TM Jr, et al. Spontaneous cervical cephalic arterial dissection and its residuum: angiographic spectrum. AJNR Am J Neuroradiol 1984;5(1):27–34.

34. Rodallec MH, Marteau V, Gerber S, et al. Craniocervical arterial dissection: spectrum of imaging findings and differential diagnosis. Radiographics 2008;28(6):1711–28.

35. Petro GR, Witwer GA, Cacayorin ED, et al. Spontaneous dissection of the cervical internal carotid artery: correlation of arteriography, CT, and pathology. AJR Am J Roentgenol 1987;148(2): 393–8.

36. Mascalchi M, Bianchi MC, Mangiafico S, et al. MRI and MR angiography of vertebral artery dissection. Neuroradiology 1997;39(5):329–40.

37. Goldberg HI, Grossman RI, Gomori JM, et al. Cervical internal carotid artery dissecting hemorrhage: diagnosis using MR. Radiology 1986;158(1): 157–61.

38. Kitanaka C, Tanaka J, Kuwahara M, et al. Magnetic resonance imaging study of intracranial vertebrobasilar artery dissections. Stroke 1994;25(3): 571–5.

39. Benninger DH, Georgiadis D, Gandjour J, et al. Accuracy of color duplex ultrasound diagnosis of spontaneous carotid dissection causing ischemia. Stroke 2006;37(2):377–81.

40. Sturzenegger M, Mattle HP, Rivoir A, et al. Ultrasound findings in carotid artery dissection: analysis of 43 patients. Neurology 1995;45(4):691–8.

41. Biffl WL, Cothren CC, Moore EE, et al. Western Trauma Association critical decisions in trauma: screening for and treatment of blunt cerebrovascular injuries. J Trauma 2009;67(6):1150–3.

42. Fusco MR, Harrigan MR. Cerebrovascular dissections: a review. Part II: blunt cerebrovascular injury. Neurosurgery 2011;68(2):517–30 [discussion: 530].

43. Schneidereit NP, Simons R, Nicolaou S, et al. Utility of screening for blunt vascular neck injuries with computed tomographic angiography. J Trauma 2006;60(1):209–15 [discussion: 215–6].

44. Mundinger GS, Dorafshar AH, Gilson MM, et al. Blunt-mechanism facial fracture patterns associated with internal carotid artery injuries: recommendations for additional screening criteria based on analysis of 4,398 patients. J Oral Maxillofac Surg 2013;71(12):2092–100.

45. Alsheik N, Gentry LR, Smoker WRK, et al. Comprehensive diagnostic evaluation of traumatic vascular injury in head trauma. Chicago (IL): RSNA; 2007.

46. Stein DM, Boswell S, Sliker CW, et al. Blunt cerebrovascular injuries: does treatment always matter? J Trauma 2009;66(1):132–43 [discussion: 143–4].

47. Cothren CC, Biffl WL, Moore EE, et al. Treatment for blunt cerebrovascular injuries: equivalence of anticoagulation and antiplatelet agents. Arch Surg 2009;144(7):685–90.

48. Lo YL, Yang TC, Liao CC, et al. Diagnosis of traumatic internal carotid artery injury: the role of craniofacial fracture. J Craniofac Surg 2007;18(2): 361–8.

49. Yang WG, Chen CT, de Villa GH, et al. Blunt internal carotid artery injury associated with facial fractures. Plast Reconstr Surg 2003;111(2):789–96.

50. Maillard AA, Urso RG, Jarolimek AM. Trauma to the intracranial internal carotid artery. J Trauma 2010; 68(3):545–7.

51. Berne JD, Reuland KS, Villarreal DH, et al. Sixteen-slice multi-detector computed tomographic angiography improves the accuracy of screening for blunt cerebrovascular injury. J Trauma 2006;60(6): 1204–9 [discussion: 1209–10].

52. Utter GH, Hollingworth W, Hallam DK, et al. Sixteen-slice CT angiography in patients with suspected blunt carotid and vertebral artery injuries. J Am Coll Surg 2006;203(6):838–48.

53. Eastman AL, Chason DP, Perez CL, et al. Computed tomographic angiography for the diagnosis of blunt cervical vascular injury: is it ready for primetime? J Trauma 2006;60(5):925–9 [discussion: 929].

54. Goodwin RB, Beery PR 2nd, Dorbish RJ, et al. Computed tomographic angiography versus conventional angiography for the diagnosis of blunt cerebrovascular injury in trauma patients. J Trauma 2009;67(5):1046–50.

55. Fakhry SM, Aldaghlas TA, Robinson L, et al. Computed tomographic angiography: false positives in the diagnosis of blunt cerebrovascular injuries. Paper presented at: American Association for the Surgery of Trauma Annual Meeting. Pittsburgh, 2009.

56. Borisch I, Boehme T, Butz B, et al. Screening for carotid injury in trauma patients: image quality of 16-detector-row computed tomography angiography. Acta Radiol 2007;48(7):798–805.

57. Levy C, Laissy JP, Raveau V, et al. Carotid and vertebral artery dissections: three-dimensional time-of-flight MR angiography and MR imaging versus conventional angiography. Radiology 1994;190(1):97–103.

58. Cothren CC, Moore EE, Ray CE Jr, et al. Carotid artery stents for blunt cerebrovascular injury: risks exceed benefits. Arch Surg 2005;140(5):480–5 [discussion: 485–6].

Pediatric Considerations in Craniofacial Trauma

Bernadette L. Koch, MD

KEYWORDS

- Pediatric craniofacial trauma • Pediatric facial fractures • Pediatric normal skull base
- Pediatric craniofacial development • Pediatric facial trauma • Toppled furniture
- All-terrain vehicle pediatric injuries • Impalement injuries

KEY POINTS

- Mechanism of injury and growth and development of the pediatric face play a role in the type and pattern of injury in pediatric craniofacial trauma.
- Normal variant lucencies in the pediatric skull base are important to recognize, so as not to misdiagnose fractures.
- Lack of complete ossification of the anterior skull base, before the age of 4 years, should not be mistaken as a posttraumatic or congenital anomaly.
- Trapdoor orbital floor fractures are more common in children than adults, and can result in entrapment of orbital soft tissues, without significant displacement of fracture fragments.
- Beware of toppled furniture, especially the television, as a cause of significant craniofacial and skull base trauma in children.
- Most pediatric craniofacial impalement injuries are treated conservatively. However, imaging is very helpful to define the extent of injury and assess for retained foreign bodies.

INTRODUCTION

Craniofacial trauma in children is in many respects very similar to that in adults. The patterns of fractures and associated injuries in older children and adolescents are frequently identical to those found in adults. However, the patterns of facial injury in younger children differ from those in adults, primarily reflecting changes in anatomy and physiology of the developing face, extent of paranasal sinus pneumatization, and phase of dentition. The frequency of different types of fractures is, therefore, also variable depending on the age of the child. In addition to understanding how normal growth and development of the pediatric skull base and craniofacial structures affect the patterns of injury in children, it is important for the imager to recognize multiple normal variant lucencies in the pediatric skull base that may mimic fractures. Furthermore, a few types of injury deserve special attention in children, including injuries related to toppled furniture, nonaccidental trauma, all-terrain vehicle (ATV) accidents, and impalement injuries.

NORMAL GROWTH AND DEVELOPMENT

Growth and development play a role in the types of craniofacial fractures that occur at differing ages. Because many of the structures are still in the process of growing and maturing, and dentition may be incomplete, pediatric maxillofacial injuries carry with them the risk of altering the function and ultimate growth of the affected structures. Therefore, timely diagnosis and prompt management are important to prevent disturbances in future growth that may affect function, dental occlusion, and cosmetic appearance. By the end of the first year of life, the mandibular halves are fused at the sympphysis. The condyle contributes to the

Disclosures and Conflict of Interests: None.
Department of Radiology, Cincinnati Children's Hospital Medical Center, University of Cincinnati College of Medicine, 3333 Burnet Avenue, Cincinnati, OH 45229, USA
E-mail address: Bernadette.koch@cchmc.org

Neuroimag Clin N Am 24 (2014) 513–529
http://dx.doi.org/10.1016/j.nic.2014.03.002

neuroimaging.theclinics.com

vertical growth of the mandible. Most growth of the zygoma and maxilla is complete by 7 years, most orbital growth is completed by 5 to 7 years of age, but cranial vault and craniofacial structures typically do not achieve growth maturity until 14 to 16 years of age.[1] The bones of the craniofacial skeleton grow and develop by remodeling and displacement throughout young life. Remodeling occurs secondary to local factors that result in change in size and shape of each component, and displacement occurs secondary to bones moving apart at joints, sutures, and articular surfaces. The cranium and orbits grow in response to the growth of the brain and globes early during the first year of life and growth of the zygoma and maxilla is initially slower than the cranio-orbital region. Therefore, the cranio-orbital complex is larger than the maxilla-mandibular complex in infancy. Over time, the young child's craniofacial development is altered by central nervous system, optic pathway, and speech/swallowing development and use and development of muscles of facial expression and mastication, paranasal sinus pneumatization, and normal phases of dentition. Deciduous teeth begin to erupt at approximately 6 months of age, mixed dentition is noted at about 6 years of age, and adult dentition is reached by 12 or 13 years of age.

Features unique to the young pediatric face that affect outcome of injury

Cranio-orbital complex is larger than the maxilla-mandibular complex in infancy

Incomplete development of the paranasal sinuses: increases stability and decreases incidence of midface fractures

Incomplete dentition: increases stability and decreases incidence of mandible fractures, rare in infants

---

NORMAL VARIANT LUCENCIES IN THE SKULL BASE

The postnatal development of the anterior and central skull base is complex, and beyond the scope of this article. The central skull base (chondrocranium) is composed of at least 25 separate ossification centers in the embryo that ultimately contribute to the mature sphenoid and occipital bones.[2] Throughout childhood, there are many normal skull base sutures, fissures, synchondroses, vascular channels, and clefts that can routinely be identified on head and neck computed tomography (CT) imaging in children. Knowledge

of the normal developmental anatomy of the skull base is important to prevent misinterpretation of these findings as fractures, osseous lesions, and cephaloceles.

A large number of normal lucencies are identified in the central skull base, including but not limited to the spheno-occipital synchondrosis, olivary eminence, craniopharyngeal canal, canalis basilaris medianus, median raphe of the basiocciput, and coronal clefts of the basiocciput. In addition, there are normal variant lucencies in the occiput that should not be confused with fractures. These include remnants of the anterior intraocciptial synchondrosis, and posterior lucencies related to variant fusion of Kerckring ossicle.

At birth, there are multiple separate ossification centers that ultimately form the mature sphenoid bone, all of which are initially separated from the adjacent centers by a nonossified synchondrosis. The most commonly visualized synchondrosis related to the sphenoid bone on postnatal CT is the spheno-occipital synchondrosis. Most skull base growth occurs at the spheno-occipital synchondrosis, which separates the postsphenoid ossification center from the basiocciput and remains patent until teenage years (**Fig. 1**). During closure, small ossified bodies may be identifiable within the spheno-occipital synchondrosis (**Fig. 2**). After closure is complete, there are frequently small divots, clefts, or fissures on one or both sides of the spheno-occipital synchondrosis.

In infants, the sphenoid body frequently contains two visible midline foramina, an anterior triangular-shaped lucency and a round posterior foramen. The anterior cartilage-containing structure is called the olivary eminence (**Fig. 3**) and is not identifiable in most older children, but may be visible as a sclerotic remnant in 11.2% of children older than 9 months of age.[2] The round posterior foramen, the craniopharyngeal canal, is a tubular lucency extending from the floor of the sella turcica to the roof of the nasopharynx (**Fig. 4**). The craniopharyngeal canal is visible on CT in 8.5% of children, and as a partial canal or sclerotic remnant in 20% of children. Rarely, this canal is pathologically widened secondary to the presence of cephaloceles that frequently contain ectopic adenohypophysis (**Fig. 5**).[3]

Most normal-variant lucencies in the occipital bone involve the basiocciput or the region of the Kerckring ossicle. Occasionally, midline lucency in the basiocciput, called the canalis basilaris medianus, is identified posterior to the spheno-occipital synchondrosis (**Fig. 6**). This structure

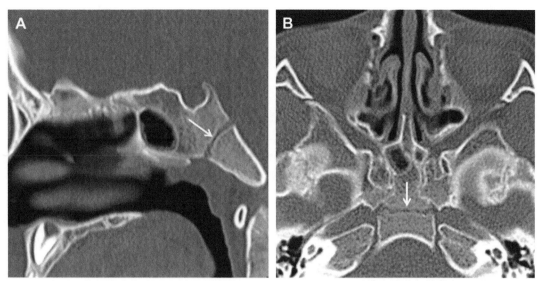

Fig. 1. Spheno-occiptal synchondrosis. (*A*) Sagittal reformatted CT image in a 4 year old demonstrates a patent spheno-occipital synchondrosis (*arrow*). (*B*) Axial bone window CT image in the same child shows the horizontal lucency between the postsphenoid and the basiocciput (*arrow*).

may be variable in shape, and complete or incomplete.[4,5] The canalis basilaris medianus is thought to represent a remnant of the cephalic end of the notochordal canal, most frequently is an incidental finding, but is rarely associated with nasopharyngeal cysts (**Fig. 7**).[5,6] The anterior intraoccipital synchondrosis has a variable appearance over time, and during fusion may progress from a somewhat cross-shaped appearance to a small well-corticated round lucency

(**Fig. 8**). Coronal clefts involving the basiocciput may also occur. Finally, lucencies related to variant fusion of Kerckring ossicle include unfused and partially fused Kerckring ossicles (**Fig. 9**), both of which, if not recognized as normal variants, may be misinterpreted as fracture. When fracture is suspected on axial imaging, three-dimensional reconstructions in these children are frequently very helpful to better define the lucencies as normal variants related to Kerckring

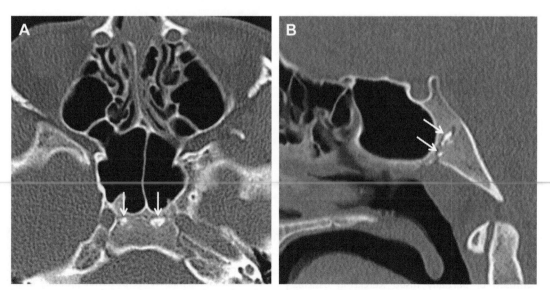

Fig. 2. Remnants of the spheno-occipital synchondrosis. (*A*) Axial and (*B*) sagittal bone window images in a 13 year old show normal variant small ossified bodies (*arrows*) within the closing spheno-occipital synchondrosis.

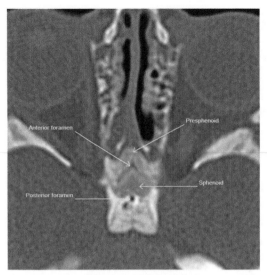

Fig. 3. Olivary eminence. Axial CT image in a 1 day old shows the typical triangular-shaped anterior foramen, called the olivary eminence, located posterior to the presphenoid and anterior to the paired main sphenoid ossification centers. This is only identifiable in infants, but may be present as a sclerotic remnant in children older than 9 months. Also easily identifiable is the posterior foramen, called the craniopharyngeal canal.

ossicle rather than fracture lines. Three-dimensional reconstructions are also helpful in proving that lucencies related to intrasutural bones, when they occur anywhere in the skull, are not fractures.

Most common normal variant sutures and lucencies in the skull base
Spheno-occipital synchondrosis: may see remnant clefts, fissures, or small ossified bodies
Olivary eminence: only identifiable in infants
Craniopharyngeal canal: floor of sella to roof of nasopharynx, completely fuses in most children, rarely contains cephalocele
Canalis basilaris medianus: usually incidental finding, rarely associated with nasopharyngeal cysts
Median raphe of the basiocciput
Coronal clefts of the basiocciput
Anterior intraocciptial synchondrosis: changes shape over time from somewhat cross-shaped to well-corticated round lucency
Unfused or partially fused Kerckring ossicle: may be confused with fracture

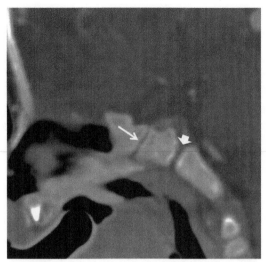

Fig. 4. Craniopharyngeal canal. Sagittal reformatted CT image in a 4-month-old child shows the normal craniopharyngeal canal (*arrow*), extending from the floor of the sella turcica to the roof of the nasopharynx, anterior to the patent spheno-occipital synchondrosis (*arrowhead*).

NORMAL ANTERIOR SKULL BASE OSSIFICATION

Imagers must also recognize several additional potential pitfalls related to the complex ossification pattern of the anterior skull base in order not to

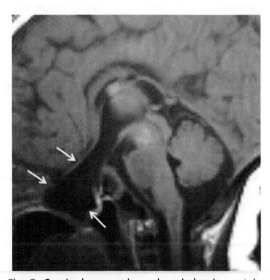

Fig. 5. Craniopharyngeal canal cephalocele containing adenohypopyhsis. Sagittal T1-weighted MR image in a 10-day-old boy demonstrates a wide, primarily cerebrospinal fluid–containing cephalocele (*arrows*), extending through the floor of the sella, into the posterior nasopharynx. Notice posterior pituitary bright spot along the dorsal aspect of the cephalocele and patent spheno-occipital synchondrosis.

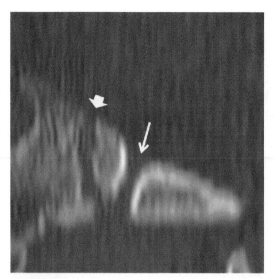

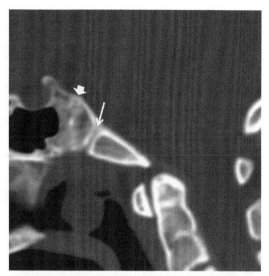

Fig. 6. Canalis basilaris medianus. Sagittal reformatted images from a temporal bone CT in a 4 year old show the patent canalis basilaris medianus (*arrow*), posterior to the patent spheno-occipital synchondrosis (*arrowhead*).

Fig. 7. Canalis basilaris medianus associated with nasopharyngeal cyst. Sagittal reformatted CT in the same child as Fig. 6, at 13 years of age, shows interval fusion of the spheno-occipital synchondrosis (*arrowhead*) and narrowing but persistent patency of the canalis basilaris medianus (*arrow*). Notice also the now visible nasopharyngeal mass just beneath the canalis basilaris medianus.

mistake such items as incomplete or multiple ossification centers as a defect from trauma, or as a cephalocele. Anterior skull base ossification occurs in a fairly predictable fashion, but with varying rates in young children. Most of the skull base at birth is composed of cartilage (Fig. 10). During the first few months of life, there is progressive ossification of the cribriform plate, roof of the nasal

cavities, and crista calli. Ossification of the cribriform plate begins near the region where the superior and middle turbinates attach and extends medially to reach the crista galli by about 2 months of age. Ossification extends from the cribriform

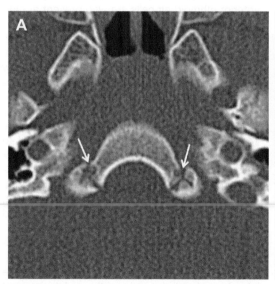

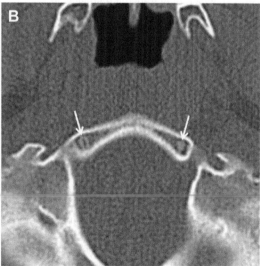

Fig. 8. Anterior intraoccipital synchondrosis. (*A*) Axial CT image in a 2 year old demonstrates somewhat cross-shaped lucencies, which represent the incompletely fused intraoccipital synchondroses (*arrows*). (*B*) Axial CT image at 7 years of age in a different child demonstrates small, foramen-like remnants of the fused intraoccipital synchondrosis (*arrows*).

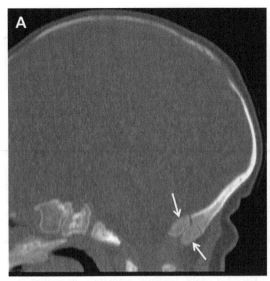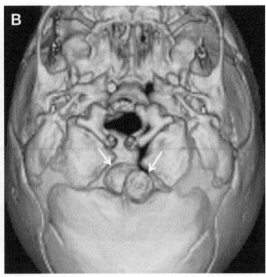

Fig. 9. Kerckring ossicle variants. (*A*) Sagittal CT in a newborn demonstrates unfused Kerckring ossicles (*arrows*). (*B*) Three-dimensional reformatted CT image in the same child demonstrates unfused duplicated Kerckring ossicles (*arrows*) at the posterior aspect of the foramen magnum.

plate, and proceeds posteriorly more quickly than anteriorly, therefore a nonossified gap is frequently present anterior to the crista galli in very young children. Only 4% of children in a study by Hughes and colleagues[7] had complete ossification of the anterior skull base by 2 years of age, whereas all patients had a fully ossified anterior skull base by the age of 3 years, 10 months (**Fig. 11**). After 4 years of age, the only unossified normal structure that remains in the midline anterior cranial fossa is the foramen cecum, just anterior to the crista galli (**Fig. 12**), which may transmit a small vein.

Anterior skull base ossification
Majority is unossified at birth
4% of children have completely ossified anterior skull base by 2 years of age
All children fully ossified anterior skull base by 4 years of age
After 4 years, only unossified portion of anterior skull basea is foramen cecum

PARANASAL SINUS DEVELOPMENT

Knowledge of normal paranasal sinus development is helpful to understand the impact and outcome of craniofacial injuries in children. For example, concern for frontal sinus fracture and its associated complications is not an issue in children who have not yet developed aeration of the frontal air cells. In addition, lack of sinus pneumatization is thought to provide increased stability

and resultant decreased incidence of midface fractures in younger children. Paranasal sinus development follows a fairly predictable pattern; however, the ultimate degree of pneumatization of each sinus is variable between individuals. The maxillary sinus is formed, but rudimentary at birth. Lateral extension of the maxillary sinus to reach the maxillary bone and inferior extension to the level of the hard palate are usually achieved by 9 years of age, with progressive pneumatization sometimes occurring until early adulthood. The anterior ethmoid air cells are also present at birth and grow until late puberty. Ethmoid pneumatization progresses in the posterior, inferomedial, and inferolateral directions until early adulthood. The sphenoid bone initially contains red marrow at birth, and conversion to fatty marrow occurs during the first 2 years of life. Subsequently, the sphenoid sinus becomes progressively pneumatized until it reaches adult size by approximately 14 years of age. The frontal sinus is the last to develop, developing from the anterior ethmoid air cells. The earliest frontal sinus pneumatization occurs around 2 years of age, by 4 years of age the frontal sinus reaches half of the height of the orbit, and by 10 years of age the frontal sinuses extend into the vertical portion of the frontal bone.[8]

Orbital fracture types vary with age, in part secondary to normal variant development of the paranasal sinuses and nasal cavities. The height of the lateral nasal wall depends on the development of the ethmoid and maxillary sinuses, and the height of the lateral nasal wall determines the height of the orbit.[9] The infant typically has relative frontal

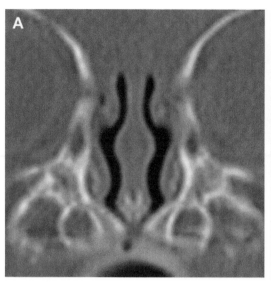 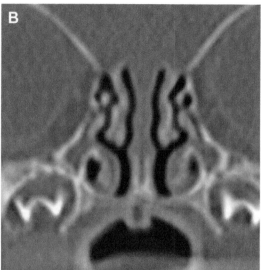

Fig. 10. Normal anterior skull base ossification at birth. (*A, B*) Coronal CT images in a newborn demonstrate the normal unossified appearance of the anterior skull.

bossing, which protects the orbital structures, but results in orbital roof fractures being more common than orbital floor fractures in the younger aged children. Furthermore, fractures of the supraorbital rim, with or without extension across the anterior cranial floor or orbital roof, are more common in younger children, and as the frontal sinuses develop, there is increased frequency of isolated frontal bone and frontal sinus fractures.[9]

Paranasal sinus development

Ethmoid sinuses present at birth, mature size by young adulthood

Maxillary sinuses present at birth, mature size by early teenage years

Sphenoid sinus absent at birth, begins development around 2 years of age, mature size by early teenage years

Frontal sinus last to develop, begins aeration at 2 years of age, mature size by early teenage years

---

DISTRIBUTION AND CAUSES OF PEDIATRIC FACIAL FRACTURES

Overall, facial fractures are less common in children than adults, with less than 15% of all facial fractures occurring in children. The lowest prevalence of pediatric facial fractures occurs in infants.[10] The prevalence of pediatric facial fractures, therefore, increases with age. There are two peaks of facial fracture, one at 6 to 7 years of age, correlating with the time when many children start attending school, and the other at 12 to 14 years of age, thought to be related to increasing physical activity and participation in sports.[10,11] In addition, there is a predominance of boys affected by facial fractures, with a ratio of up to 8.5:1.[10,12] The primary causes of pediatric facial fractures in descending order of frequency are motor vehicle accidents; sports-related injury; and accidental causes, such as falls, and violence.[12]

The frequency of different types of facial fractures in children varies in the literature, with most studies showing that mandible and nasal fractures are the most common, followed by maxillary/zygoma fractures. Although nasal fractures are common, septal hematomas remain rare, but of significant importance because when they occur, they require immediate surgical drainage to prevent septal cartilage necrosis, saddle nose deformity, and, in the young child, midface growth retardation.[10] The low incidence of mandible fractures in children younger than the age of 4 years is thought to be secondary to the relative increase in strength of the mandible at this age, which is at least in part secondary to the presence of unerupted dentition. Incomplete dentition, with tooth buds still present within the maxilla and mandible, provides stability and resistance to fracture. In addition, children are thought to be relatively resistant to facial fractures because of more flexible suture lines, greater elasticity/flexibility of the osseous structures of the face, and a thicker layer of protective subcutaneous fat typically present in the pediatric face.[10,12]

When mandibular fractures occur in children, they are more likely to be unilateral fractures than in their adult counterparts. In children younger

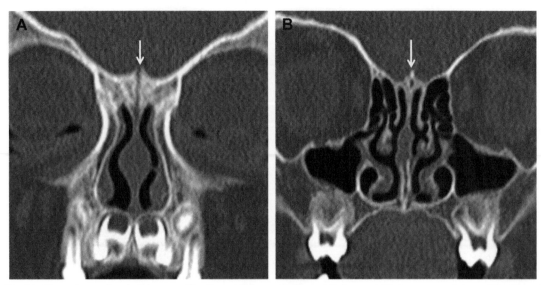

Fig. 11. Normal anterior skull base ossification at 2.5 years of age. (*A*) Coronal CT shows complete ossification of the anterior skull base with the exception of visible margins of the foramen cecum (*arrow*). (*B*) Coronal CT in the same child, 1 cm posterior to the foramen cecum, shows complete ossification of the floor of the anterior cranial fossa, on either side of the crista galli (*arrow*).

than 6 years of age, condylar fractures are typically intracapsular, whereas in older children they are more commonly extracapsular and involve the condylar neck. Subcondylar fractures with a greenstick fracture of the mandibular neck are common in children. CT imaging with multiplanar reconstruction and three-dimensional reformatted images are helpful in identifying mandible fractures in the young child, because many of the fracture lines are difficult, if not impossible, to see on conventional radiographs (Fig. 13).

Orbital floor fractures may be simple or comminuted and may occur as an isolated fracture or in association with other facial fractures. Orbital floor fractures are rare in children younger than the age of 5 years, increase in frequency as children get older, and do not exceed upper orbit fractures in frequency until after the age of 7.1 years.[13] In

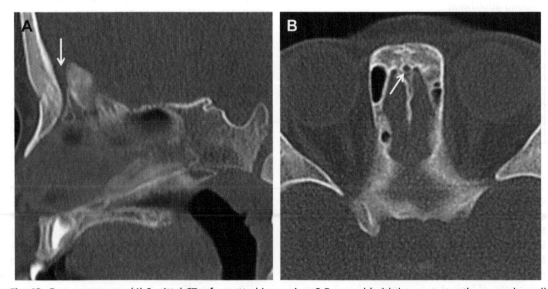

Fig. 12. Foramen cecum. (*A*) Sagittal CT reformatted image in a 2.5-year-old girl demonstrates the normal, small unossified foramen cecum (*arrow*), anterior to the ossified crista galli. (*B*) Axial CT images demonstrate the tiny, well-defined round remnant of unossified foramen cecum (*arrow*).

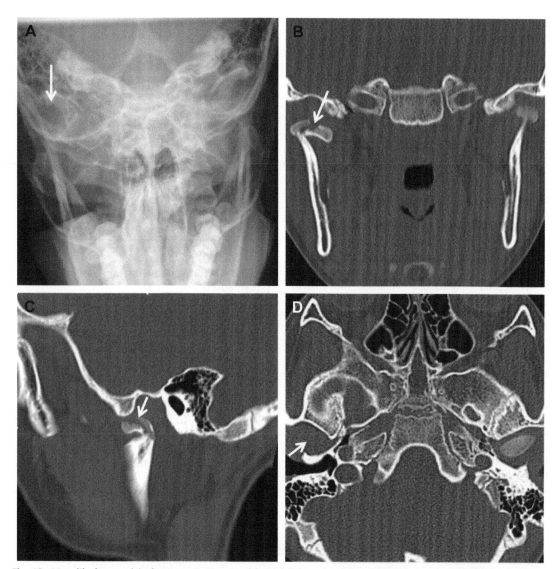

Fig. 13. Mandibular condyle fracture. A 13-year-old girl fell from her bike and has jaw pain with decreased range of motion. (*A*) Towne view from a mandibular radiograph series shows a more lucent right condylar fossa (*arrow*) when compared with the left, but no definite fracture (oblique mandible films were suboptimal in positioning and are not shown). (*B*) Coronal and (*C*) sagittal bone window reformatted CT images in the same child clearly demonstrate a comminuted right mandibular condyle fracture (*arrows*) with anterior and medial displacement of fragments out of the condylar fossa. (*D*) Axial CT bone window image at the level of the condylar fossa demonstrates the empty condylar fossa on the right (*arrow*). Care must be taken not to miss this finding, which may be the only indication of mandibular condyle fracture on axial head CT.

1957, Smith and Regan[14] first described a blowout fracture as one in which the orbital floor was fractured, but not the infraorbital rim. This is typically the result of a blow to the orbit by an object that is larger than the bony orbit, with the force absorbed by the orbital rim and transmitted to the orbital walls. The inferior and medial walls are most susceptible to fracture. With increased pressure on the intraorbital contents, there is a resultant "blowout" of the fractured inferior or medial orbital walls. A pure orbital floor blowout fracture spares the inferior orbital rim, whereas an impure blowout fracture involves the inferior orbital rim. In the original report, patients presented with diplopia, enophthalmos, paresthesia in the distribution of the infraorbital nerve, and soft tissue injury. In older children and adults, orbital floor fractures are most commonly secondary to interpersonal altercations or motor vehicle accidents, but younger children usually sustain orbital floor fractures related to accidents, such as falls, and sporting injuries.[15] A particular type of orbital floor fracture that occurs in children more frequently than adults is the trapdoor fracture. This is a linear, hinged, orbital floor fracture that occurs secondary to relatively deficient mineralization of the orbital floor. If the minimally displaced fracture fragment springs back into its normal position it may cause entrapment of intraorbital soft tissues and/or extraocular muscle (**Fig. 14**). This may result in ischemia and necrosis; may lead to fibrosis and scarring; and may be responsible for persistent diplopia, even after surgical correction. In addition, the trapdoor fracture may be associated with oculocardiac reflex, which may cause headache, nausea and vomiting, bradycardia, and potential syncope. When this occurs, urgent surgical correction is indicated.[16,17] Despite the presence of restricted extraocular muscle movement, external signs of swelling and ecchymosis may be minimal, and therefore this has also been termed the "white-eyed blowout fracture."[18]

The overall goal of treatment of craniofacial fractures in children is the same as adults (ie, to re-establish anatomy and function back to the preinjury state). However, the specific timing and choice of treatment may vary depending on the age of the child with respect to how much future residual growth is predicted, and the overall phase of dentition at the time of injury.[10,19] Children in general have greater osteogenic potential and heal faster, therefore anatomic reduction may be accomplished earlier and necessary immobilization times may be shorter. However, fracture immobilization and fixation may be more difficult than in adults, depending on the stage of dentition. For various reasons, deciduous teeth may not be ideal for placement of fixation devices, and care must be taken not to injure intraosseous tooth buds and erupting teeth while trying to place fixation screws and plates.[10]

A few specific causes of craniofacial trauma in children deserve special attention, namely trauma secondary to toppled furniture, inflicted injury/child abuse, injuries related to ATV accidents, and impalement injuries.

Distribution of pediatric facial fractures
Facial fractures much less common in children than adults
Lowest prevalence of pediatric facial fractures occurs in infants
Two peaks in prevalence of pediatric facial fractures: 6 to 7 years and 12 to 14 years of age
Predominance of boys affected by pediatric facial fractures, up to 8.5:1 boys/girls
Mandible and nasal bone fractures more common than maxillary/zygoma fractures
Unilateral mandibular fractures more common in children than adults
Trapdoor orbital floor fracture more common in children than adults

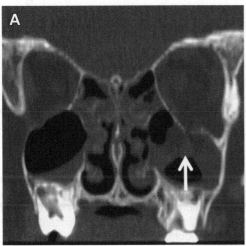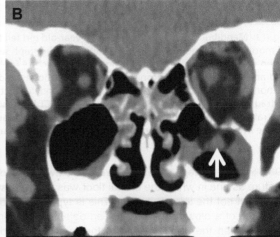

Fig. 14. Trapdoor orbital floor fracture. A 5 year old involved in an ATV accident, with complete inability to move the left eye upward. (*A*) Coronal reformatted bone window orbit CT image shows a minimally displaced left orbital floor fracture with mixed attenuation material extending into the superior left maxillary sinus (*arrow*). (*B*) Coronal reformatted soft tissue window image at the same level clearly defines the inferior rectus muscle (*arrow*) and fat herniated into the upper maxillary sinus.

TOPPLED FURNITURE

Much has been published in the literature on the topic of pediatric injuries related to toppled furniture.[20–29] These are almost universally preventable injuries and therefore there have been many attempts by the medical community and manufacturers to educate the consumer, with warning labels about securing furniture with appropriate straps and wall mounts, and recommendations about appropriate television stands. Despite these attempts, childhood injury from tipover or toppled furniture is a significant problem, and because of the weight of toppled furniture relative to small children, injuries can be severe and sometimes fatal. Televisions and clothes dressers/armoires are frequently the offending agents, and televisions placed on top of dressers, chests, or armoires account for nearly half of all injuries related to toppled televisions.[21,24,26]

Many years ago, cathode ray tube televisions were bulky and difficult to tip over. More recent changes in television construction have resulted in continued increase in pediatric injury related to toppled television. The flat-panel television sets

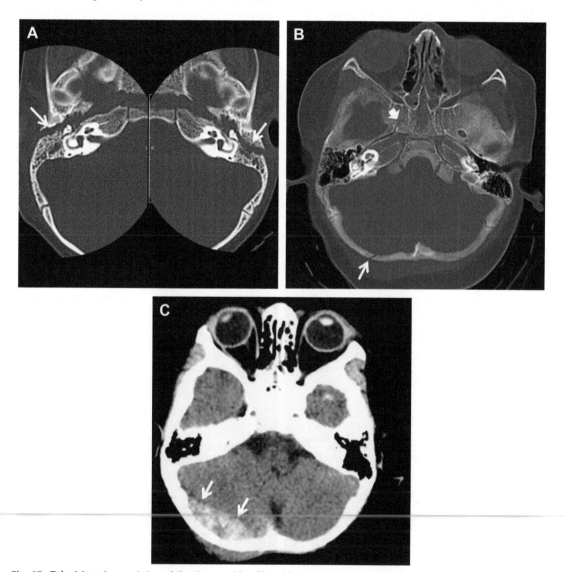

Fig. 15. Television tipover injury. (*A*) A 3 year old suffered fatal head injury secondary to 22-inch television falling on her head. Axial temporal bone CT demonstrates widely diastatic bilateral temporal bone fractures (*arrows*). (*B*) A 2-year-old boy was climbing on a dresser that supported a television when the television fell and landed on the child's head. Axial bone window CT images demonstrate nondisplaced fractures of the right occiput (*arrow*) and sphenoid base (*arrowhead*). (*C*) Axial soft tissue CT image in the same child as in *B* better identifies a lenticular-shaped high-attenuation venous epidural hematoma (*arrows*).

are larger and more slender in shape, frequently have a narrow base with a center of gravity that is more toward the front of the television, and are rarely secured to the object on which they rest. Televisions are reportedly present in 96.7% of households in the United States, and children reportedly watch more than 28 hours per week of television.[28] This incredibly frequent exposure to a television provides innumerable opportunities for children to suffer from television-related injuries, particularly because children understandably do not recognize the danger of climbing on unstable furniture. In a large-scale 22-year study by De Roo and colleagues, 17,313 children required emergency treatment of television-related injuries each year, and the rate of injury attributable to falling televisions increased by 95% over the 22-year period. The median age of patients was 3 years and 64.3% of patients were younger than 5 years. Lacerations and soft tissue injuries were most common but concussions and closed head injuries represented 13.3% of injuries among children younger than 5 years and 7.7% of injuries among patients aged 11 to 17 years.[30] Murray and coworkers[25] reported 42,122 injuries and found the injury rate to be highest for children 1 to 4 years of age; most injuries in that group of children involved the head and neck. Television-related crush injury frequently results in calvarial and skull base fractures, including involvement of the orbital roofs, sphenoid bone, and temporal bones (**Fig. 15**).[22,23,27] Mortality rates from television tipover injuries are reported between 1.9% and 20%, depending on the series,[20,24] with most deaths occurring in children younger than 3 years of age secondary to traumatic brain injury.[20]

NONACCIDENTAL, INFLICTED TRAUMA, AND CHILD ABUSE

Mandibular fractures are exceedingly uncommon in infants. When mandibular fractures do occur in infants, unilateral fractures are more common than bilateral fractures. Because they are so uncommon, recognition of such injury should at least raise suspicion for a direct blow related to child abuse, particularly if the mechanism of reported injury is incongruous with the resultant fracture.[19,31,32] In addition, because infants are unable to verbalize jaw pain, and signs of external trauma may be lacking, imagers should be sure to inspect the mandibular condyles and condylar fossa on head CTs performed for evaluation of suspected child abuse, because fractures of the mandibular condyle, with or without displacement of the condyle into the middle cranial fossa, may be clinically silent in young patients (**Fig. 16**).

ATV ACCIDENTS

With increasing popularity of ATV use comes an increase in ATV-related accidents, with an

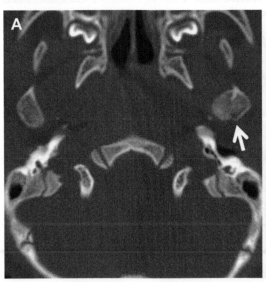
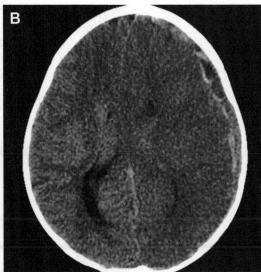

Fig. 16. Mandibular condyle fracture secondary to fatal nonaccidental trauma. (*A*) Axial bone window CT image obtained for evaluation of a 9 month old who was found down, with blown pupils, demonstrates a mildly displaced left mandible condyle fracture (*arrow*). (*B*) Axial soft tissue head CT image shows a large, mixed attenuation left-sided subdural hematoma with significant left-to-right shift of midline structures, and diffuse hypodensity and ill-definition of the left cerebral hemisphere gray-white differentiation consistent with hypoxic/ischemic injury. This unfortunate child also sustained parietal and occipital bone fractures and splenic and liver lacerations (not shown).

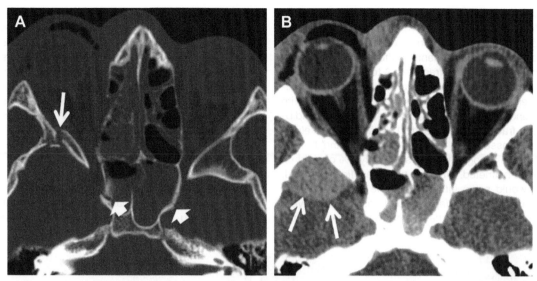

Fig. 17. ATV facial fractures. (*A*) Axial bone window CT image in a teenager who suffered craniofacial and intracranial trauma in an ATV accident shows fractures of the right greater sphenoid wing (*arrow*) and bilateral sphenoid sinus walls (*arrowheads*) with associated preseptal soft tissue gas and subtotal opacification of the ethmoid and sphenoid sinuses. (*B*) Axial soft tissue window CT image in the same patient shows to better advantage the associated right preseptal orbital soft tissue swelling and the right middle cranial fossa epidural hematoma (*arrows*). This child unfortunately sustained multiple additional sites of facial fracture and intracranial hemorrhage, in addition to bilateral carotid artery dissections and right cavernous-carotid fistula (images not included). (*Courtesy of* Carl Pergam, MD, Tucson, AZ.)

associated increase in pediatric craniofacial trauma (**Fig. 17**). A total of 40% of all ATV-related fatalities occur in pediatric patients, and many of these children die from head and neck injuries. Prigozen and coworkers[33] reviewed 26 children with a mean age of 13.1 years with craniofacial injuries secondary to ATV accidents. A total of 65% of them were drivers of the ATV. Injuries most frequently occurred secondary to loss of control/rollover accidents, falls from the vehicle, and collision with stationary objects. Fractures of the facial bones and skull occurred in 77%. Midface injuries

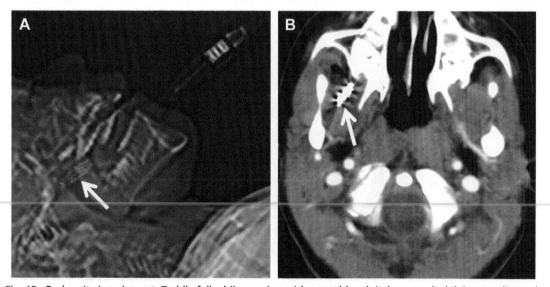

Fig. 18. Oral cavity impalement. Toddle fell while running with a toothbrush in her mouth. (*A*) Scout radiograph from face CT shows the toothbrush protruding from the child's mouth with the bristles of the brush overlying the oropharynx (*arrow*). (*B*) Axial soft tissue CT image clearly shows the bristle portion of the brush (*arrow*) embedded within the right masticator space with surrounding soft tissue gas. (*Courtesy of* Carl Pergam, MD, Tucson, AZ.)

were the most common and isolated craniofacial fractures of mandible, maxilla, nasal, or orbital bones were uncommon, occurring in only 20% of patients. Most patients suffered two or more concomitant facial fractures. A total of 35% of children had closed head injuries, and in these children, there was a significant association with mandible fractures. Patients sustaining mandibular fractures were nearly 13 times more likely to have associated closed head injury and tended to have a longer hospital stay. Only 8% of children were helmeted. Although not scientifically proved, it would seem intuitive that the use of helmets, particularly with face protection, would prevent many of these injuries. There have been multiple efforts by the medical community to educate consumers and dealers about the dangers of riding ATVs, and there have been increasing regulations with respect to ATV use. However, many parents and children fail to follow the recommended injury prevention measures, and therefore there has been a continued increase in the number of injuries and deaths in children involved in ATV-related accidents in recent years.[34–36]

IMPALEMENT INJURIES

Impalement injuries involving the oral cavity in children are common, especially in toddlers who fall while carrying objects in their mouth, most

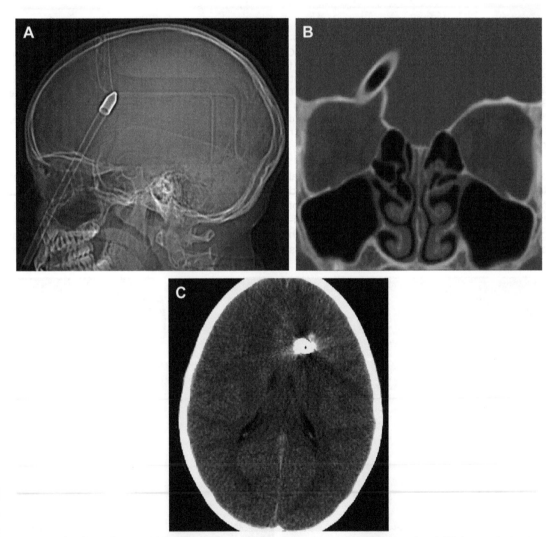

Fig. 19. Orbital impalement with intracranial extension. (A) Scout radiograph from head CT demonstrates a radiodense distal end of an arrow on which this 8 year old impaled his orbit. (B) Coronal bone window CT image shows to better advantage the trajectory of the hollow plastic shaft of the arrow traversing the fractured orbital roof. (C) Axial soft tissue window head CT image clearly shows the tip of the arrow within the contralateral left frontal lobe.

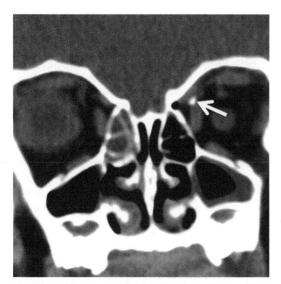

Fig. 20. Orbital impalement with retained intraorbital pencil graphite. A 5 year old fell on a pencil, had upper eyelid puncture wound, and suspicion of retained pencil fragments. Coronal soft tissue window CT image shows high-attenuation graphite fragment (*arrow*) along the superior margin of the left medial rectus muscle. In addition, there is extraconal soft tissue swelling, edema, and hemorrhage superior to the fragment, inseparable from the superior oblique muscle.

commonly sticks, writing instruments, toothbrushes (**Fig. 18**), cylindrical toys, and straws. Most children sustain injury to the palate, posterior oropharynx, tonsillar region, or cheek, with fewer injuries involving the tongue and floor of mouth.

Most patients are treated conservatively, without complications, and only a minority of patients requires imaging.[37–39] Matsusue and coworkers[38] reviewed 144 children with oral cavity impalement injury. The impaled objects were toothbrushes in 20.8%, cylindrical toys in 18.8%, and chopsticks in 13.2%. The soft palate was involved in 44.4% and the hard palate was involved in 18.1%. CT examination was performed in 11.1%, admission was required in only 8.3%, most healed spontaneously or with minimal intervention, and there were no complications of deep infection or neurologic sequelae. However, there are occasional reports of complications, such as deep neck infection, life-threatening hemorrhage, internal carotid artery thrombosis, mediastinitis, and airway complications.[39–42]

Occasionally with oral cavity injuries, and frequently with other craniofacial impalement injuries (particularly those involving neck and orbit), the entrance wound is the only site of clinically evident trauma and imaging may be necessary to determine trajectory of the puncture injury and the total extent of injury (**Fig. 19**). Furthermore, imaging is helpful in children (and adults) who have sustained an impalement injury when there is suspicion of retained foreign body, for instance when the offending object is broken and the missing piece cannot be located (**Fig. 20**). CT is the primary imaging modality of choice in these patients, to identify the path of penetration, the presence or absence of retained foreign body, and any associated craniofacial fractures and/or intracranial

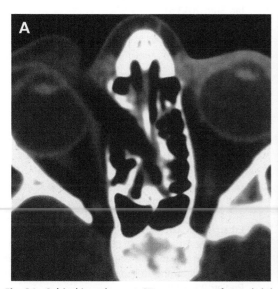
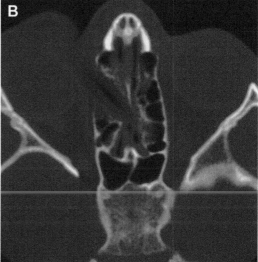

Fig. 21. Orbital impalement CT appearance of wood. (*A*) Axial soft tissue window CT image of an 11-year-old boy who fell on a twig, demonstrates a large linear orbital foreign body of air attenuation, deviating the globe laterally and traversing the left ethmoid air cells. (*B*) Axial bone window CT image at the same level demonstrates the periphery of the twig to be soft tissue attenuation and the central portion air attenuation.

injury.[43] Wood foreign bodies, such as remnants of twigs or pencils, may be particularly difficult to recognize, because early on they may have the attenuation of air (Fig. 21), becoming intermediate in attenuation and inseparable from surrounding soft tissues as they absorb moisture.[44–47] In addition, the CT appearance depends on the window/level setting at which the image is viewed.

SUMMARY

When comparing craniofacial trauma in children with adults, there are several differences, primarily related to the mechanisms of injury and timing of the injury with respect to the normal growth and development of the pediatric face and skull base. Older children and adolescents are more similar to adults with respect to mechanism of injury and distribution of facial fractures, whereas younger children have a lower incidence of facial fractures and different distribution of fractures when they do occur. The lack of paranasal sinus pneumatization and presence of incomplete dentition impart a relative increased strength to the osseous structures of the pediatric face. The difference in size of the craniofacial ratio and relative frontal bossing in young children also contribute to the pattern of facial fractures in children. A few specific causes of craniofacial trauma in children are of particular interest, including injuries related to toppled furniture, nonaccidental trauma, ATVs, and those secondary to craniofacial or neck impalements.

REFERENCES

1. Costello BJ, Rivera RD, Shand J, et al. Growth and development considerations for craniomaxillofacial surgery. Oral Maxillofac Surg Clin North Am 2012; 24(3):377–96.
2. Madeline LA, Elster AD. Postnatal development of the central skull base: normal variants. Radiology 1995;196(3):757–63.
3. Abele TA, Salzman KL, Harnsberger HR, et al. Craniopharyngeal canal and its spectrum of pathology. AJNR Am J Neuroradiol 2014;35(4):772–7.
4. Currarino G. Canalis basilaris medianus and related defects of the basiocciput. AJNR Am J Neuroradiol 1988;9(1):208–11.
5. Morabito R, Longo M, Rossi A, et al. Pharyngeal enterogenous cyst associated with canalis basilaris medianus in a newborn. Pediatr Radiol 2013;43(4): 512–5.
6. Lohman BD, Sarikaya B, McKinney AM, et al. Not the typical Tornwaldt's cyst this time? A nasopharyngeal cyst associated with canalis basilaris medianus. Br J Radiol 2011;84(1005):e169–71.
7. Hughes DC, Kaduthodil MJ, Connolly DJ, et al. Dimensions and ossification of the normal anterior cranial fossa in children. AJNR Am J Neuroradiol 2010; 31(7):1268–72.
8. Scuderi AJ, Harnsberger HR, Boyer RS. Pneumatization of the paranasal sinuses: normal features of importance to the accurate interpretation of CT scans and MR images. AJR Am J Roentgenol 1993;160(5):1101–4.
9. Cobb AR, Jeelani NO, Ayliffe PR. Orbital fractures in children. Br J Oral Maxillofac Surg 2013;51(1):41–6.
10. Zimmermann CE, Troulis MJ, Kaban LB. Pediatric facial fractures: recent advances in prevention, diagnosis and management. Int J Oral Maxillofac Surg 2005;34(8):823–33.
11. Imahara SD, Hopper RA, Wang J, et al. Patterns and outcomes of pediatric facial fractures in the United States: a survey of the National Trauma Data Bank. J Am Coll Surg 2008;207(5):710–6.
12. Alcala-Galiano A, Arribas-Garcia IJ, Martin-Perez MA, et al. Pediatric facial fractures: children are not just small adults. Radiographics 2008;28(2):441–61 [quiz: 618].
13. Koltai PJ, Amjad I, Meyer D, et al. Orbital fractures in children. Arch Otolaryngol Head Neck Surg 1995; 121(12):1375–9.
14. Smith B, Regan WF Jr. Blow-out fracture of the orbit; mechanism and correction of internal orbital fracture. Am J Ophthalmol 1957;44(6):733–9.
15. Egbert JE, May K, Kersten RC, et al. Pediatric orbital floor fracture: direct extraocular muscle involvement. Ophthalmology 2000;107(10):1875–9.
16. Gerber B, Kiwanuka P, Dhariwal D. Orbital fractures in children: a review of outcomes. Br J Oral Maxillofac Surg 2013;51(8):789–93.
17. Sires BS, Stanley RB Jr, Levine LM. Oculocardiac reflex caused by orbital floor trapdoor fracture: an indication for urgent repair. Arch Ophthalmol 1998; 116(7):955–6.
18. Jordan DR, Allen LH, White J, et al. Intervention within days for some orbital floor fractures: the white-eyed blowout. Ophthal Plast Reconstr Surg 1998;14(6):379–90.
19. Goth S, Sawatari Y, Peleg M. Management of pediatric mandible fractures. J Craniofac Surg 2012;23(1): 47–56.
20. Gokhan S, Kose O, Ozhasenekler A, et al. Mortality and morbidity in children caused by falling televisions: a retrospective analysis of 71 cases. Int J Emerg Med 2010;3(4):305–8.
21. Gottesman BL, McKenzie LB, Conner KA, et al. Injuries from furniture tip-overs among children and adolescents in the United States, 1990-2007. Clin Pediatr 2009;48(8):851–8.
22. Jea A, Ragheb J, Morrison G. Television tipovers as a significant source of pediatric head injury. Pediatr Neurosurg 2003;38(4):191–4.

23. Marnewick J, Dansey R, Morreau P, et al. Television tip-overs: the Starship Children's Hospital experience and literature review. Injury 2011;42(5):534–8.

24. Muniz AE. Craniofacial injuries from television tip-over. Pediatr Emerg Care 2012;28(1):52–4.

25. Murray KJ, Griffin R, Rue LW III, et al. Recent trends in television tip over-related injuries among children aged 0-9 years. Inj Prev 2009;15(4):240–3.

26. Rutkoski JD, Sippey M, Gaines BA. Traumatic television tip-overs in the pediatric patient population. J Surg Res 2011;166(2):199–204.

27. Yahya RR, Dirks P, Humphreys R, et al. Children and television tipovers: a significant and preventable cause of long-term neurological deficits. J Neurosurg 2005;103(Suppl 3):219–22.

28. AC Nielsen Company. Television audience report 2010 & 2011. Available at: http://www.nielsen.com/content/dam/corporate/us/en/reports-downloads/2011-Reports/2010-2011-nielsen-television-audience-report.pdf. Accessed January 7, 2014.

29. US Consumer Product Safety Commission. Product instability or tip-over injuries and fatalities associated with televisions, furniture, and appliances: 2012 report. Available at: www.cpsc.gov/PageFiles/135118/tipover2012.pdf. Accessed January 7, 2014.

30. De Roo AC, Chounthirath T, Smith GA. Television-related injuries to children in the United States, 1990–2011. Pediatrics 2013;132(2):267–74.

31. Knoche JW, LeBlanc KK, King TW, et al. An infant with a unilateral mandibular fracture: when to consider nonaccidental trauma. Clin Pediatr 2012;51(4):404–7.

32. Schlievert R. Infant mandibular fractures: are you considering child abuse? Pediatr Emerg Care 2006;22(3):181–3.

33. Prigozen JM, Horswell BB, Flaherty SK, et al. All-terrain vehicle-related maxillofacial trauma in the pediatric population. J Oral Maxillofac Surg 2006;64(9):1333–7.

34. Brann M, Mullins SH, Miller BK, et al. Making the message meaningful: a qualitative assessment of media promoting all-terrain vehicle safety. Inj Prev 2012;18(4):234–9.

35. Shah SR, McKenna C, Miller M, et al. Safety factors related to all-terrain vehicle injuries in children. J Trauma Acute Care Surg 2012;73(4 Suppl 3):S273–6.

36. Mangano FT, Menendez JA, Smyth MD, et al. Pediatric neurosurgical injuries associated with all-terrain vehicle accidents: a 10-year experience at St. Louis Children's Hospital. J Neurosurg 2006;105(Suppl 1):2–5.

37. Hellmann JR, Shott SR, Gootee MJ. Impalement injuries of the palate in children: review of 131 cases. Int J Pediatr Otorhinolaryngol 1993;26(2):157–63.

38. Matsusue Y, Yamamoto K, Horita S, et al. Impalement injuries of the oral cavity in children. J Oral Maxillofac Surg 2011;69(6):e147–51.

39. Younessi OJ, Alcaino EA. Impalement injuries of the oral cavity in children: a case report and survey of the literature. Int J Paediatr Dent 2007;17(1):66–71.

40. Chauhan N, Guillemaud J, El-Hakim H. Two patterns of impalement injury to the oral cavity: report of four cases and review of literature. Int J Pediatr Otorhinolaryngol 2006;70(8):1479–83.

41. Kosaki H, Nakamura N, Toriyama Y. Penetrating injuries to the oropharynx. J Laryngol Otol 1992;106(9):813–6.

42. Kupietzky A. Clinical guidelines for treatment of impalement injuries of the oropharynx in children. Pediatr Dent 2000;22(3):229–31.

43. Pereira KD, Wang BS, Webb BD. Impalement injuries of the pediatric craniofacial skeleton with retained foreign bodies. Arch Otolaryngol Head Neck Surg 2005;131(2):158–62.

44. Adesanya OO, Dawkins DM. Intraorbital wooden foreign body (IOFB): mimicking air on CT. Emerg Radiol 2007;14(1):45–9.

45. Pyhtinen J, Ilkko E, Lahde S. Wooden foreign bodies in CT. Case reports and experimental studies. Acta Radiol 1995;36(2):148–51.

46. Uchino A, Kato A, Takase Y, et al. Intraorbital wooden and bamboo foreign bodies: CT. Neuroradiology 1997;39(3):213–5.

47. Yamashita K, Noguchi T, Mihara F, et al. An intraorbital wooden foreign body: description of a case and a variety of CT appearances. Emerg Radiol 2007;14(1):41–3.

Surgical Perspectives in Craniofacial Trauma

Paul J. Schmitt, MD[a,*], Dane M. Barrett, MD[b], J. Jared Christophel, MD[c,d], Carlos Leiva-Salinas, MD[e], Sugoto Mukherjee, MD[e], Mark E. Shaffrey, MD[a]

KEYWORDS

- Neuroimaging • Craniofacial trauma • Traumatic brain injury • Surgical management

KEY POINTS

- The craniofacial skeleton and the associated viscera and soft tissue encompass a range of systems, all serviced by different medical and surgical specialists.
- Patients with traumatic injuries involving craniofacial anatomy will often require multidisciplinary management, and prioritizing their multiple problems is critical to providing efficient and effective care.
- Radiologists who are familiar with some of the chief concerns of the surgeons that manage this anatomically diverse region can help expedite the decision-making process by keeping some of these concerns in mind when they report their findings.

Learning Objectives

1. Review the primary imaging modalities used for assessing craniofacial trauma.
2. Review the mechanisms behind the various injuries seen in craniofacial trauma patients.
3. Discuss craniofacial injuries that require surgical management.
4. Discuss elements of craniofacial imaging studies that are critical to the surgeon for surgical planning and decision-making.

INTRODUCTION

The key to understanding the radiologic evaluation of craniofacial trauma is through a thorough knowledge of anatomy and mechanisms of traumatic injury. Craniofacial anatomy is diverse. Bony elements include the anterior skull vault, skull base, and the facial skeleton. The viscera contained in the craniofacial skeleton consist of the frontal lobes, orbital contents, segments of all the cranial nerves, the upper airway, and the digestive tract. In addition to the individual components, structural areas must be assessed as a whole. As a result of this anatomic diversity, physicians from numerous different specialties

---

Disclosures: The authors have no disclosures or conflicts of interest to report.

[a] Department of Neurological Surgery, University of Virginia Health System, PO Box 800212, Charlottesville, VA 22908, USA; [b] Department of Otolaryngology-Head and Neck Surgery, University of Virginia Health System, PO Box 800713, Charlottesville, VA 22908, USA; [c] Division of Head & Neck Surgical Oncology, Department of Otolaryngology-Head and Neck Surgery, University of Virginia Health System, PO Box 800713, Charlottesville, VA 22908, USA; [d] Division of Facial Plastic & Reconstructive Surgery, Department of Otolaryngology-Head and Neck Surgery, University of Virginia Health System, PO Box 800713, Charlottesville, VA 22908, USA; [e] Division of Neuroradiology, Department of Radiology and Medical Imaging, University of Virginia Health System, PO Box 800170, Charlottesville, VA 22908, USA

* Corresponding author.

E-mail address: PJS5Y@virginia.edu

Neuroimag Clin N Am 24 (2014) 531–552

http://dx.doi.org/10.1016/j.nic.2014.03.007

neuroimaging.theclinics.com

scrutinize similar imaging sets, although looking for very different pathologic abnormalities within the same anatomic regions. A well-run trauma center can convey relevant pathologic abnormality to the appropriate services with speed, accuracy, and efficiency. It is important to have a firm understanding of injuries representing a surgical emergency versus those that may be more appropriate for less urgent intervention. The elements of imaging studies most relevant to the surgeon managing a craniofacial trauma patient are discussed.

ANATOMY
Visceral Anatomy

Patients who present with a history and physical examination suggestive of a severe head injury should undergo initial evaluation with a noncontrast head computed tomography (CT), particularly if there is any neurologic deficit or airway compromise. Common screening strategies that direct decision-making for CT evaluation include the New Orleans Criteria[1] and the Canadian Head CT Rule.[2–4] Although a routine CT will adequately screen for major injuries and intracranial pathologic abnormality, more dedicated studies may be indicated to help characterize the nature of the patients' injuries. Patients who have suspected or known facial fractures should undergo further imaging using thinner slices through the face, using both bone and soft tissue algorithms.

The craniofacial viscera are imaged in the acute trauma setting with CT. If there is an indication for further imaging, specifically with respect to the intracranial contents and the globes, a magnetic resonance (MR) imaging is typically obtained at a later time. An MR imaging protocol for a craniofacial trauma patient should include T1 and T2 weighted sequences, fluid attenuated inversion recovery (FLAIR), susceptibility weighted imaging (SWI) or gradient echo (GRE), and diffusion-weighted imaging (DWI) sequences, with scans acquired in the axial, coronal, and sagittal planes. Typically, the information gleaned from an MR image is not used in determining immediate surgical indications. However, information obtained on an MR image may help clarify a presentation that is not explained by CT findings alone. Such information may, for example, determine whether a patient needs intracranial pressure monitoring.

MR imaging becomes especially helpful in cases of severe traumatic brain injury, or when patients have undergone or will undergo a decompressive procedure. If the degree of axonal and neuronal damage is so severe that a significant recovery is not likely, it could impact the willingness of both the surgeon to operate and the family to consent to a procedure. Although decompressive craniectomies can be lifesaving, it is important for family members to have realistic expectations regarding a patient's long-term outcome; information provided by GRE/SWI and DWI in the acute and subacute periods can help the surgeon set realistic recovery goals (Fig. 1). Thus, "heroic" procedures may not be offered given additional negative prognostic findings on the MR study.

Vascular Anatomy

Vascular anatomy of the craniofacial region includes the carotid arteries and vertebrobasilar circulation, as well as the venous drainage of the head and neck. Direct evidence of, or mechanisms of injury suggesting (eg, distracting injuries), vascular injury should always be considered on initial imaging, even though noncontrast CT is not the proper imaging modality for such a diagnosis (Fig. 2). Injury to the carotid canal, sella turcica, or dural venous sinuses should prompt further evaluation with a dedicated vascular study, such as CT or MR angiography (CTA and MRA, respectively), or digital subtraction angiography (DSA). CTA and MRA both have various strengths and weaknesses. In general, CTA is often more practical in the trauma setting, because it is a quicker study to obtain, and it is more widely available. CTA typically involves a submillimeter overlapping axial acquisition, and a rapid bolus contrast injection using a vessel tracking technique.[5,6] If there is a high likelihood of an indication for intervention, the patient may be taken directly for a DSA, which can also provide a possible venue for endovascular treatment of some vascular injuries.

Skeletal Anatomy

The craniofacial skeleton is typically evaluated with a submillimeter data set, reconstructed at 1 to 3 mm in the axial, coronal, and sagittal planes. It is useful to consider the facial buttress system when evaluating the craniofacial skeleton (Fig. 3). The facial buttress system is divided into vertical and horizontal buttresses, with the vertical buttresses absorbing the bulk of the force generated during mastication. The vertical buttresses consist of paired medial, lateral, and posterior buttresses, as well as a single midline buttress. Horizontal buttresses are present in each facial-third connecting and reinforcing the lateral buttresses. The facial buttresses generally correlate with ideal lines of osteosynthesis and are thus an important consideration in facial plating. Accurate knowledge of the fracture pattern and how it impacts the facial buttress system guides the craniofacial surgeon in appropriate restoration of form and function.

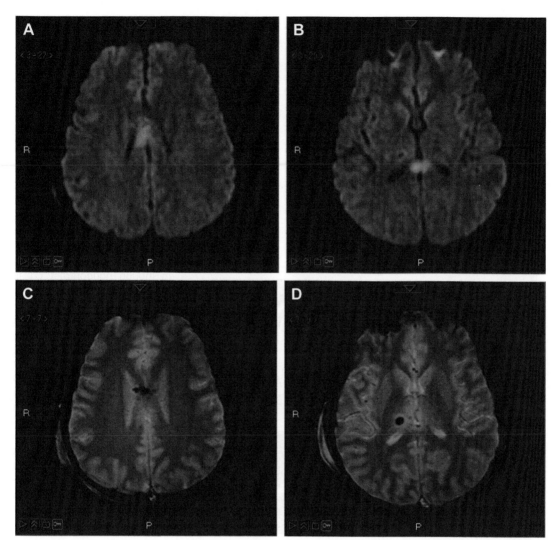

Fig. 1. Diffuse axonal injury. Typical MR imaging findings associated with DAI, which results from shear stress at points of relative fixation as manifested by areas of restricted diffusion in the body (*A*) and splenium (*B*) of the corpus callosum. Note the presence of blood on gradient echo sequences in the body of the corpus callosum (*C*). Additional areas of hemorrhagic DAI are seen in the right thalamus (*D*).

IMAGING FINDINGS

Plain films no longer play a significant role in evaluating craniofacial trauma. Patients with outward signs of facial trauma should have a noncontrast head CT on arrival in the hospital. Assessment of imaging should be systematic and comprehensive. A useful scheme is to assess the intracranial contents first for overt pathologic abnormality. Next, the soft tissues should be examined for signs of trauma, because this will direct attention to scrutinize other structures in that area, and along the same line of force that may be impacted. Next, the bony structures are assessed, starting superficially with the cranial vault, orbits (**Box 1**), nasal bones (**Box 2**), and sinuses (**Box 3**), then moving attention to the deeper structures and the skull base (**Box 4**).

Critical in the initial evaluation of head CT studies in trauma is the search for intracranial hemorrhage and mass effect, followed by evaluation for more subtle findings. After the intracranial contents have been thoroughly assessed, the bony elements are evaluated. The radiologist should keep fracture patterns in mind, along with frequently missed areas, such as the lamina papyracea, orbital rims and floor, nasolacrimal duct,

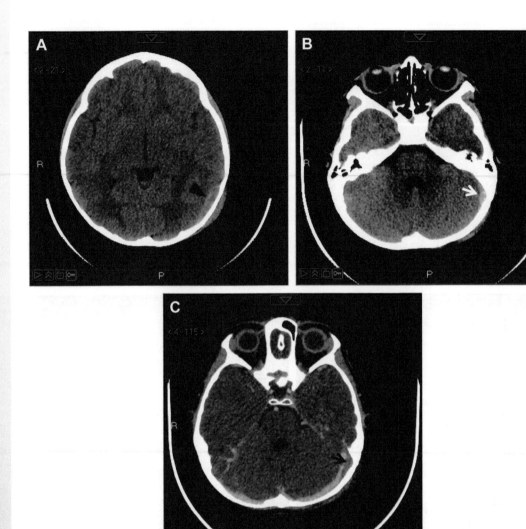

Fig. 2. This 3-year-old patient fell from a laundry cart and landed on the back of her head. She was found to have an epidural hematoma (*black arrowhead in A*) and an associated thrombus of the left transverse and sigmoid sinuses. The thrombus is seen as a hyperdensity in the noncontrast study in (*white arrow in B*) and as a filling defect in the CT venogram (*black arrow in C*).

carotid canal, temporal bones, and orbital apex. The radiologist should conclude with the occipital condyles, C1 and C2 vertebrae and the rest of the craniocervical junction, and the skull base. Based on initial findings, further studies may be recommended, such as dedicated imaging of the facial bones or sinuses, angiographic studies, and/or MR imaging.

PATHOLOGIC ABNORMALITY
Cranial Injuries

Cranial injuries can be categorized broadly into soft tissue, bony, and hemorrhagic injuries. The soft tissue of the cranium is essentially limited to the scalp. As such, diagnosis of injury here is not heavily reliant on imaging, with the possible exception of detection of foreign bodies. Although a growing subgaleal hematoma could require surgical intervention, such a problem should readily manifest itself on a physical examination. Skull fractures are discussed later with injuries to the craniofacial skeleton.

Hemorrhagic injuries
Hemorrhagic injuries are grouped into intra-axial and extra-axial lesions. Intra-axial blood is confined to the parenchyma, whereas extra-axial

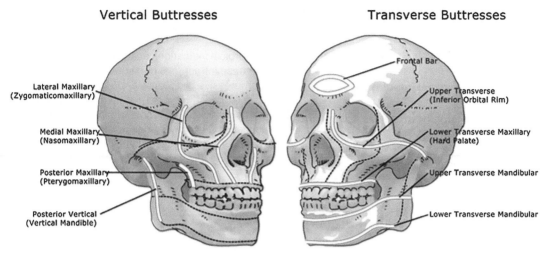

Fig. 3. The lateral vertical (zygomaticomaxillary) buttress extends from the inferolateral maxilla at the malar eminence along the lateral orbital rim to the frontal bone. The medial (nasomaxillary) buttress extends along the medial maxilla, borders the piriform aperture, and ends superiorly into the frontal bone. The posterior (pterygomaxillary) buttress extends along the posterior maxilla and pterygoid plates to the skull base. The midline buttress consists of the vomer and perpendicular plate of the ethmoid and connects the palatine process of the maxilla to the frontal bone.[35] The horizontal buttresses occur across the frontal bone, below the orbits, above and below the teeth, across the palate, and along the bottom of the mandible.

blood can be found anywhere in the ventricles or in the spaces between the calvarium and the cortex. Most of the traumatic hemorrhagic pathologic abnormalities can have atraumatic analogues that may change further diagnostic testing and management indications. Although the clinical history will typically clarify such an ambiguity, there are frequently cases where the causality between a hemorrhage and a trauma is not clear. For instance, a fall down a flight of stairs could result in traumatic subarachnoid hemorrhage; likewise, an aneurysm that ruptures in a patient who is

walking down a flight of stairs could also cause a fall but would also have subarachnoid hemorrhage of a disparate cause. Patients are also frequently "found down," and the volume of hemorrhage on a head CT may be out of proportion to a ground level fall. Noting discrepancies between the size of a given hemorrhage, and the absence of other signs of trauma, such as soft tissue injuries, skull fractures, and contrecoup injuries (**Fig. 4**), can help the trauma team and surgeons initiate appropriate management algorithms. In these instances, MR imaging is often useful for assessing diffuse

---

Box 1
Pearls for diagnosis of orbital fractures

- Identify any grossly abnormal globe position
- Quantify the size of the fracture defect
- Assess the integrity of the lamina papyracea
- Identify involvement of the infraorbital canal
- Evaluate for orbital fat herniation, and comment on volume, as high-volume herniation contributes to entrapment
- Compare the ocular muscles on each side to assess for contusion
- Evaluate for globe injury
- In children, assess for trapdoor fractures

Box 2
Pearls for diagnosis of nasal bone fractures

- Differentiate high and low defects from fractures
- Look for soft tissue swelling or other local evidence of trauma to determine fracture acuity
- Most fractures will occur in the transverse plane
- Crossing the plane of the nasal bone differentiates the nasociliary groove from a fracture
- Look for involvement of the maxilla
- Determine if there is an associated NOE or midface fracture
- Inspect the septum for swelling or deviation to diagnose septal hematoma

axonal injury (DAI) and other subtle findings that may be difficult to identify on CT.

Intra-axial injury

Intra-axial injury can take the form of intracerebral or intracerebellar hematomas (**Fig. 5**), edema, contusions, and DAI. Both cortical contusions and intracerebral hematomas are the result of impact disrupting the vessels supplying the area of injury. If there is sufficient force, the injury at the impact site—or "coup" injury—may have a contrecoup sibling injury (see **Fig. 4**). Although a coup injury is the result of direct impact, contrecoup injuries are a result of the acceleration forces generated in areas of brain parenchyma that are distant from the impact point.[7] Although common viewpoints are that coup and contrecoup injuries must be categorized along the same line of force, this is not actually the case.

The rotational acceleration underlying contrecoup lesions may also cause the microhemorrhages indicating severe DAI, depending on the mechanism of impact. Microhemorrhages occur when sheer stress injures the small vessels at points of the neuraxis joining a relatively mobile structure with one that is fixed. Anatomic sites especially prone to microhemorrhages include

the corpus collosum, centrum semiovale, periventricular white matter, and the brainstem (see **Fig. 1**).

Surgical indications arise when these conditions increase intracranial pressure, necessitating a decompressive procedure and/or evacuation. DAI is not of great concern in the acute period. As mentioned earlier, widespread hemorrhagic or ischemic DAI may influence the decision to intervene surgically at a later date in a patient's hospital course, as it is a poor prognostic factor.

Extra-axial injuries

Extra-axial hemorrhage occurs in the subdural, epidural, subarachnoid, or intraventricular spaces. Intraventricular hemorrhage will rarely occur in isolation, and when it does, atraumatic causes should be explored. Subdural hematomas can occur when bridging veins between the dura and the arachnoid are disrupted (**Fig. 6**). This disruption can occur as a result of direct impact, but is more commonly due to inertia. Elderly people are especially susceptible to subdural hematomas, because cortical atrophy places greater stress on the bridging veins. Subdural hematomas are not bound by dural attachments and thus may cover the entire convexity.

Epidural hematomas are usually associated with a skull fracture at the site of hemorrhage; the fracture fragments tear a dural artery or vein and the blood will collect in the epidural space. Because epidural blood will be contained by dural attachments to the skull, these will typically have a lenticular shape and will have significant mass effect and sulcal effacement (**Fig. 7**). Epidural bleeding is most commonly arterial, but it can be venous as well.

For epidural and subdural bleeding, the volume of hemorrhage and/or degree of mass effect is often used as a metric for surgical intervention. Furthermore, evidence of active bleeding, such as a "swirl sign," could indicate the need for an emergent evacuation (see **Fig. 7**).

Traumatic subarachnoid hemorrhage is not always an indication for surgery or even advanced imaging, provided the referring clinicians are confident that the cause is trauma and not a vascular event. If there is any question as to the cause of the hemorrhage, the patient should be sent for vascular imaging. When there is a discrepancy between the mechanism of injury and the pattern of hemorrhage, there should be a low threshold for vascular imaging, because failure to treat aneurysmal bleeding or a ruptured arteriovenous malformation can have devastating consequences. Nonaneurysmal subarachnoid hemorrhage is not trivial, despite the lack of indication for

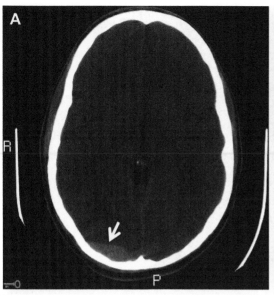
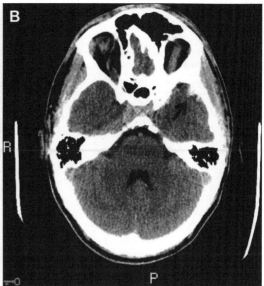

Fig. 4. An example of coup-contrecoup injury. Note the epidural hematoma (*white arrow in A*), and the associated contusion in the left temporal pole (*black arrow in B*). Epidural hematomas are frequently associated with a contrecoup injury, although the lesion may not be as obvious as it is here.

intervention, as it has been shown to be an independent predictor of poor outcomes.[8] It is, however, important to distinguish it from aneurysmal subarachnoid hemorrhage to prevent unnecessary and expensive vascular diagnostic studies, given the additional issues of radiation and contrast nephropathy.

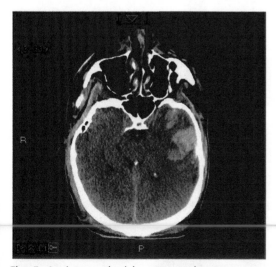

Fig. 5. An intracerebral hematoma due to trauma. The superficial location of the hemorrhage, the presence of additional findings of calvarial and skull base fractures, along with history of trauma help in making the correct diagnosis. It is important to look for, and comment on, associated injuries to neighboring structures, which may favor traumatic cause.

Surgical management of traumatic brain injury
Common guidelines for surgical intervention combine radiologic findings with the patient's mental status and overall clinical condition. The Brain Trauma Foundation Guidelines[9–12] for the surgical management of various hemorrhagic conditions are outlined in Table 1. Although the more detailed statistics may not necessarily be of great importance to the radiologist, the nature of the radiological criteria should be taken into careful consideration. Accurate documentation of findings, such as degree of midline shift, volume of hemorrhage, or the change in one of those metrics between serial studies, can help surgeons in their decision-making process. A commonly used method for quickly calculating hemorrhage volume is the ellipsoid, or "ABC method,"[13] described in Fig. 8.

Vascular Injuries

Vascular injury should be included in the differential diagnosis of every patient presenting with craniofacial injuries. Dissections, pseudoaneurysms, and arteriovenous fistulae almost always require intervention, be it surgical or medical (Figs. 9 and 10). CTA is a fast and reliable screening tool in patients who have findings suspicious for a vascular cause, or who have injuries that predispose them to a vascular injury. Although standard DSA provides both diagnostic and therapeutic opportunities, a DSA requires the patient undergo a relatively lengthy procedure

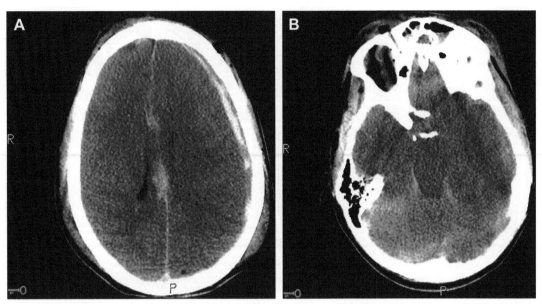

Fig. 6. An example of traumatic subdural hematoma. The blood seen in (*A*) clearly crosses dural attachments, as it covers the entire left convexity. In this case, there was significant mass effect, resulting in uncal herniation and complete effacement of the basal cisterns, seen in (*B*).

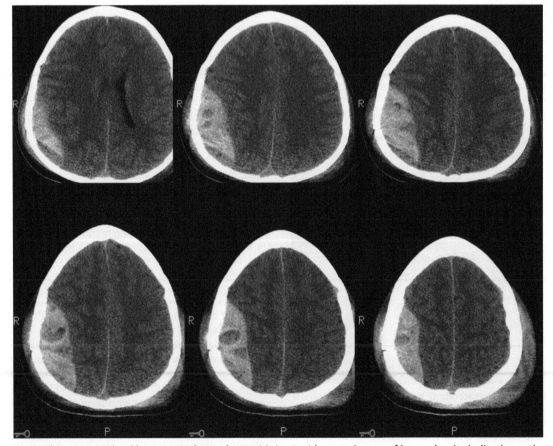

Fig. 7. This acute epidural hematoma shows the "swirl sign" with central areas of lower density indicating active bleeding. There is less mass effect seen with an epidural hematoma than there is with a subdural hematoma of comparable volume.

Table 1
The Brain Trauma Foundation guidelines for the surgical management of various hemorrhagic conditions

Pattern of Hemorrhage	Indications for Surgical Management
Epidural	Volume >30 cm³ GCS <9 with focal neurologic deficit

Subdural	>10-mm thickness
	>5-mm midline shift
	GCS <9 *AND*:
	  2-point drop in GCS since initial injury
	  OR
	  Fixed/dilated or asymmetric pupils
	  OR
	  ICP >20 mm Hg

Intracerebral	Volume >50 cm³
	Medically refractory ICP
	Neurologic deterioration
	Volume >20 cm³ *AND*:
	  >5-mm midline shift
	  OR
	  Cisternal effacement

Posterior fossa	Evidence of mass effect:
	  Distortion of the fourth ventricle
	  OR
	  Effacement of the basal cisterns
	  OR
	  Obstructive hydrocephalus

Abbreviation: GCS, Glasgow Coma Scale.
Data from Refs.[9–12]

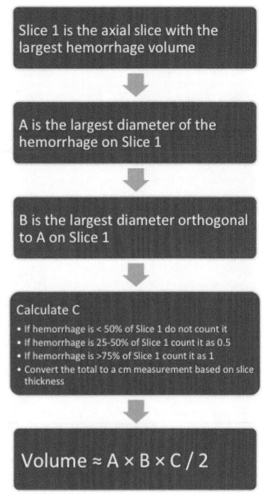

Slice 1 is the axial slice with the largest hemorrhage volume

↓

A is the largest diameter of the hemorrhage on Slice 1

↓

B is the largest diameter orthogonal to A on Slice 1

↓

Calculate C
- If hemorrhage is < 50% of Slice 1 do not count it
- If hemorrhage is 25-50% of Slice 1 count it as 0.5
- If hemorrhage is >75% of Slice 1 count it as 1
- Convert the total to a cm measurement based on slice thickness

↓

$$Volume \approx A \times B \times C / 2$$

Fig. 8. Flowchart for using the "ABC" or ellipsoid method for calculating the volume of a hematoma on CT.

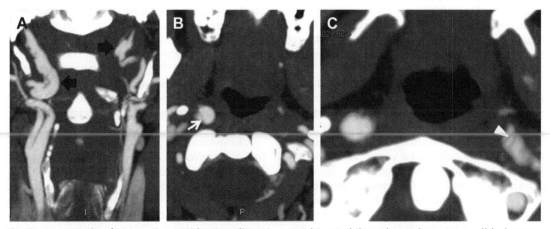

Fig. 9. An example of traumatic carotid artery dissections resulting in bilateral pseudoaneurysms (*black arrows in A*). The dissection flaps within the right (*white arrow in B*) and left (*white arrowhead in C*) carotid arteries are depicted nicely in axial views.

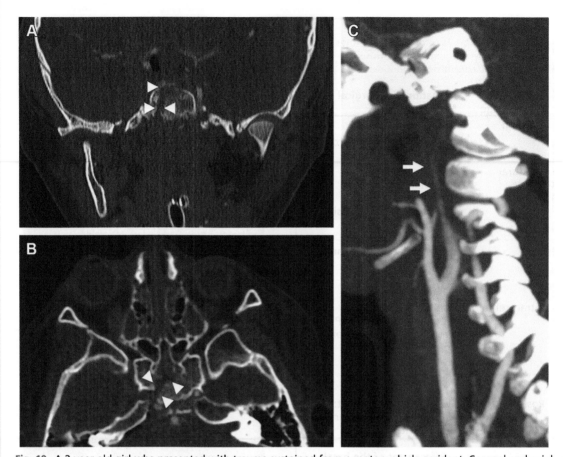

Fig. 10. A 2-year-old girl who presented with trauma sustained from a motor vehicle accident. Coronal and axial noncontrast facial CT images (*A, B*) show oblique fractures through the central skull base extending across the nonpneumatized sphenoid bone, clivus, and sellar floor, with mild displacement of fragments (*arrowheads*). The fracture line traverses the sphenoid bone and extends into the right carotid canal and petroclival fissure (*arrowheads in B*). Sagittal CTA neck image (*C*) shows decreased opacification with reduced caliber of the cervical segment of the right internal carotid artery, compatible with traumatic dissection (*arrows in C*).

compared with CTA. Unless there is the potential for life-saving therapy, the length of the procedure may prove prohibitive in an unstable patient. Given the advancements in availability, technique, and reliability of CTA studies, DSA for all practical purposes is reserved for a minority of patients.

A dissection refers to a tear in the wall of a vessel, resulting in the formation of an intramural hematoma. The dissection flap is sometimes seen in axial views on a CTA or MRA (see **Fig. 9**), although its absence does not rule out dissection. A change in the caliber of a vessel, vessel occlusion, and an intraluminal thrombus are also signs of a traumatic dissection. Pseudoaneurysms occur when there is a complete disruption of the vessel wall, resulting in a hematoma. The wall of the pseudoaneurysm is formed by the hematoma; thus, it is not a true aneurysm. Treatment of dissections with or without resultant pseudoaneurysms depends on

the presence of symptoms, and the location of the dissection. First-line therapy is medical management with either antiplatelet or anticoagulant therapy. There have been no randomized controlled trials comparing the 2 modalities, and reported nonrandomized trials have not found one to be superior to the other.[14–16] Patients who are symptomatic despite medical management, or in whom a dissection fails to resolve, may be indicated for endovascular management with stenting and/or coiling.

Arteriovenous fistulae occur when an injured artery communicates directly with a venous space. The carotid-cavernous fistula (CCF) is a type of arteriovenous fistula that results from the cavernous carotid or carotid artery branches emptying into the cavernous sinus. The Barrow classification stratifies CCFs by the type of arterial feeders (**Table 2**).[17] Traumatic CCFs are usually direct (type A). These CCFs result from a

Table 2
The Barrow classification

Type	Flow	Arterial Source
A	High	ICA
B	Low	ICA meningeal branches
C	Low	ECA meningeal branches
D	Low	ICA and ECA meningeal branches

Data from Barrow DL, Spector RH, Braun IF, et al. Classification and treatment of spontaneous carotid-cavernous sinus fistulas. J Neurosurg1985;62(2):248–56. http://dx.doi.org/10.3171/jns.1985.62.2.0248.

communication between the cavernous carotid and the cavernous sinus. Indirect CCFs (type B–D) are fed by external carotid artery (ECA) and/or internal carotid artery (ICA) branches. Fractures of the sphenoid bone and the adjacent bones of the central skull base predispose patients to developing CCF (**Fig. 11**). Traumatic CCFs rarely thrombose spontaneously and are usually embolized endovascularly (see **Fig. 11**). Failure to treat a direct CCF can result in visual loss, due to elevated intraorbital pressure from reversal of blood flow into the orbit. Engorgement of intraorbital veins, specifically the superior ophthalmic vein, should raise suspicion of a

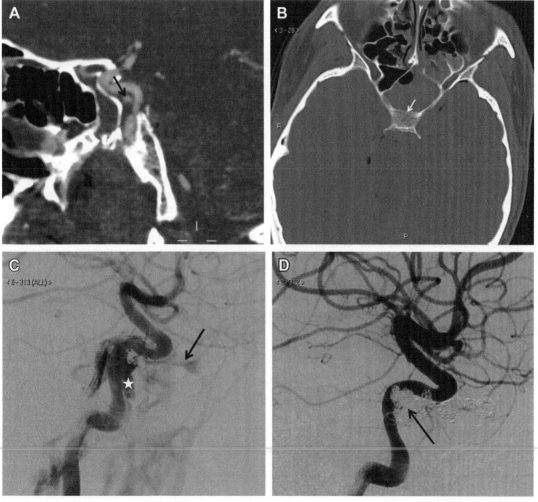

Fig. 11. Direct (Barrow type A) CCF. This patient was noted to have contrast extravasation from the cavernous carotid on a CT angiogram (*black arrow in A*), which was in proximity to a sellar fracture (*white arrow in B*). Such fractures are commonly associated with CCFs. DSA confirms the fistula with contrast outside the cavernous carotid within the cavernous sinus (*white star in C*) as well as extending into the superior ophthalmic vein (*black arrow in C*). Postembolization DSA shows complete resolution with no evidence of any contrast within the cavernous sinus along with coils in the cavernous sinus (*black arrow in D*).

CCF. Although a CCF can sometimes be diagnosed or suspected on a routine study such as CTA or MRA, optimal and precise evaluation frequently requires a mutiphasic CTA (arterial and venous phases), MRA/MR venogram, or a DSA. DSA has the added therapeutic advantage of potentially treating the fistula at the same time.

Skeletal Injuries

Bony injury to the craniofacial skeleton may be managed by observation, closed reduction, or open reduction and internal fixation. Optimal open reduction and internal fixation of the craniofacial skeleton involve plating fractures across lines of ideal osteosynthesis. Semirigid techniques have proven to be more effective in the craniofacial skeleton compared with the rest of the bony skeleton. These techniques rely on the use of small plates and screws that allow micromotion across fracture lines, resulting in secondary bone healing. Accurate assessment of the bony craniofacial injuries guides the type, timing, and method of intervention.

Skull fractures

Skull fractures can occur because of blunt force or a penetrating injury. Fractures are often described as linear, depressed, compound, or some combination of the 3 fractures. Linear fractures typically result from force distributed over a large area. Depressed fractures, on the other hand, require a great deal of force be focused on a small area of the skull, to deform and fracture the point of impact. Compound fractures may be linear or depressed, but involve a direct communication with the external environment. Linear fractures can be managed with expectant observation. Serial imaging is necessary to ensure that the fracture is not growing, because a growing fracture would be an indication for surgical management. Depressed skull fractures are surgically reduced if the depressed fragment is displaced by a distance greater than the thickness of the skull. However, smaller depressions may be managed surgically for cosmetic reasons, if they are in a prominent area such as the forehead. The management of penetrating injuries is typically conservative, especially when the missiles project intracranially. Local debridement of devitalized tissue is advocated over aggressive measures to retrieve foreign bodies.

Frontal sinus fractures

Frontal sinus fractures are relatively uncommon fractures of the craniofacial skeleton, and when present, typically occur in association with other facial fractures.[18] Fractures involving the frontal sinus invariably tear the internal mucosal lining,

resulting in hemorrhage, which allows easy exclusion of frontal sinus fractures when free fluid is not present within the sinus during the acute phase.[19] When a fracture is present, there are several key radiographic findings that influence surgical management. These findings include the presence of an anterior table fracture, a posterior table fracture, a fracture involving the nasofrontal recess, and the presence of a dural tear.

When a fracture of the frontal sinus is present, two-thirds of cases involve the anterior table only. Surgical repair of isolated anterior table fractures is considered in the setting of esthetic deformity, which depends on the degree of fracture displacement. Minimally displaced fractures can generally be observed.

Posterior table fractures are prone to more significant morbidity and are often associated with cerebrospinal fluid (CSF) leaks, meningitis, traumatic brain injury, and long-term mucocele formation. The degree of posterior table displacement and amount of pneumocephalus are important radiographic findings influencing surgical decision-making. Minimally displaced posterior table fractures (less than 2 mm or width of the table) are typically observed unless a persistent CSF leak develops.[20] Comminuted fractures and those associated with more significant fracture displacement (greater than 2 mm or width of the table) are more frequently associated with dural tear and frank CSF leak and generally require repair with neurosurgical assistance. The status of frontal sinus outflow tract (FSOT) should be assessed as obstruction of this tract can result in mucocele formation and is best assessed in the sagittal plane (**Fig. 12**).

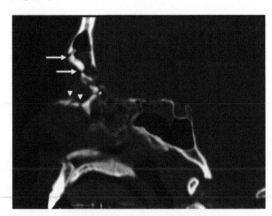

Fig. 12. A 45-year-old woman involved in a motor vehicle accident as an unrestrained driver. Sagittal noncontrast facial CT images show fracture of the nasal bones (*arrowheads*) and anterior wall of the frontal sinuses (*arrows*). Fracture is disrupting the sinus drainage (*asterisk*) and can predispose for a frontal sinus mucocele.

Nasal bone fractures

Fractures of the nasal bones are the most common fractures involving the craniofacial skeleton, and one of the most common fractures in adults.[21,22] Eighty percent of nasal fractures occur below the intercanthal line, where the nasal bones are thinnest. Diagnosing nasal bone fractures is not always straightforward. It is common to confuse a suture line for a fracture and versa fracture for a suture line. It is helpful to remember that nasal fractures are typically oriented in the transverse plane and can cross midline (Fig. 13). Sutures and nasociliary grooves, however, are longitudinally oriented and do not cross midline. Associated clinical symptoms, adjacent soft tissue swelling, and availability of prior studies for comparison are helpful in confounding cases.

The primary goals for treatment of nasal bone fractures are restoration of cosmesis and nasal airflow. The treatment options consist of observation as well as closed or open reduction techniques with or without septoplasty. Although imaging is not necessary for diagnosis and management of nasal bone fractures, when available, it may influence management. During imaging review, it is important to ensure there is not associated ethmoid involvement. Attention must also be given to the cartilaginous structures of the nose, which are often injured in conjunction with nasal bone fractures. Concurrent septal fractures are associated with failure of closed reduction treatment and therefore may influence surgical decision-making if present.[23]

Fractures of the cartilaginous septum can result in perichondrial separation and hematoma formation. Hematomas may compromise the blood supply to the cartilage, resulting in necrosis, infection, and saddling of the nasal dorsum in the long term. In addition to assessing the nasal bones, it is vital for the radiologist to assess the septum for swelling or traumatic deviation. The presence of a septal hematoma requires prompt intervention to avoid the long-term complications of septal perforation or sclerotic septal distortion, which may compromise nasal airflow.

Naso-orbital-ethmoidal fractures

More severe blows to the central face may involve not only the nasal bones but also the ethmoid sinuses and medial orbital rims. Referred to as naso-orbital-ethmoid (NOE) fractures, this fracture pattern disrupts the confluence of the medial maxillary buttress with the upper transverse maxillary buttress (Fig. 14). The anterior nasal structures will commonly be displaced posteriorly into the lacrimal bones and ethmoid sinuses with splaying of the medial orbital walls and globe malposition. Telecanthus, or increased distance between the medial orbital walls, is the hallmark finding.

NOE fracture patterns are classified by the status of the central medial orbital wall and medial canthal tendon. Type I fractures consist of a large bone fragment attached to the medial canthal tendon. Type II fractures involve medial canthal tendon attachment to smaller comminuted fragments. Type III fractures involve complete avulsion of the medial canthal tendon.[24,25] Grading of the fracture pattern is often best made by physical examination or intraoperatively, although 3-dimensional reformatting may provide clues as to which type of fracture pattern is present.

It is important for both the radiologist and the craniofacial traumatologist to assess the status of the FSOT in the presence of NOE fractures. Traumatic injury of the FSOT may result in adhesions, obstruction, and mucocele formation. If the outflow tract is involved, frontal sinus obliteration may be necessary.

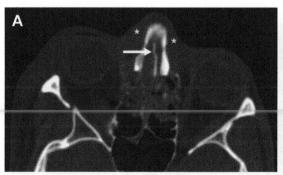
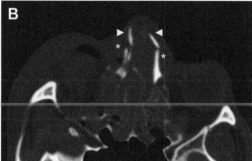

Fig. 13. A 26-year-old man involved in a motor vehicle accident as an unrestrained driver. Axial noncontrast facial CT images (*A, B*) show fracture of the nasal septum (*arrow in A*) and comminuted fracture of the nasal bones (*arrowheads in B*). Note the soft tissue swelling/hematoma surrounding the nasal bones (*asterisks*). The patient was also noted to have a right orbital blow-out fracture involving the right zygomaticosphenoid fissure and the orbital floor.

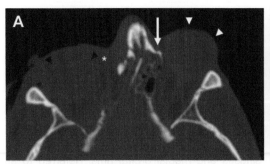
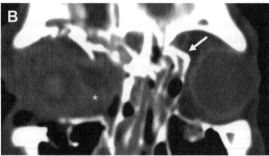

Fig. 14. A 32-year-old man involved in a motor vehicle accident as a restrained driver with a left NOE fracture and bilateral medial orbital fractures. Axial (*A*) and coronal (*B*) noncontrast facial CT images show posterior and left lateral displacement of the bony nose and left ethmoid structures resulting in a lateral displacement of the left medial orbital wall (*white arrows in A and B*) causing proptosis (*white arrowheads in A*). The lamina papyracea is displaced medially on the right, expanding the orbital volume and causing right enophthalmos (*A, black arrowheads*). Note the increased distance between the medial right orbital wall and the medial aspect of the right globe with associated hemorrhage surrounding the medial canthal ligament (*asterisk*), concerning for ligamentous injury.

Injuries to the orbit and orbital contents

Orbital "blow-out" fractures are purely internal fractures involving the medial wall and/or orbital floor without involvement of the orbital rim. A direct blow to the orbit can transmit energy through the rim to the thinner orbital floor and lamina papyracea resulting in an orbital blow-out fracture (**Fig. 15**).

Herniation of orbital contents into the maxillary sinus confirms an orbital floor fracture. Fractures of the medial wall or lamina papyracea can be quite subtle. Orbital emphysema in the absence of an obvious orbital fracture is suggestive of a medial wall fracture. In more obvious cases, orbital fat and medial rectus muscle may be displaced medially. Fractures of either the floor or the medial wall may result in increased orbital volume and subsequent enophthalmos.

Surgical intervention is geared toward correcting diplopia secondary to entrapment and preventing enophthalmus. Entrapment should be suspected whenever there is herniation of orbital fat or muscle through the medial wall or orbital floor. Kinking of the herniated muscle through the fracture increases suspicion of entrapment. Often, the herniated muscle will have a more rounded appearance characterized by a 1:1 height-to-width ratio, indicating disruption of the fascial sling and an increase in the likelihood of entrapment and late enophthalmus.[26] Involvement of more than 50% of the orbital floor and greater than 2 mm of soft tissue prolapse into the maxillary and ethmoid sinuses are also indications for repair.[27] Both the radiologist and the surgeon should be attuned to these factors during imaging review.

Orbital roof fractures frequently occur in conjunction with frontal sinus and skull base fractures. Associated findings include pneumocephalus, dural tears, CSF leaks, intracranial

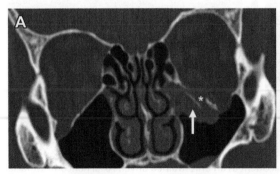
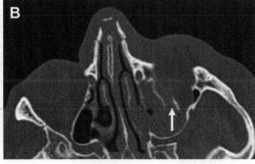

Fig. 15. A 29-year-old man involved in a fight, with a direct blow to the left orbit. Coronal (*A*) and axial (*B*) noncontrast facial CT images show inferior blowout fracture of the left orbit. There is inferior displacement of the left orbital floor (*arrow*) with herniation of intraorbital fat and a small amount of extraconal hemorrhage along the inferior rectus muscle (*asterisk*).

hemorrhage, and meningoencephaloceles. Orbital roof fractures often demonstrate inferior displacement of fracture fragments into the orbit and are thus also termed "blow-in" fractures. A major risk of "blow-in" fractures is ocular injury, which is thought to occur with greater incidence than the 2% to 23% reported in all orbital fracture types.[28–30]

Orbital apex fractures are rare. When identified, it is vital to exclude retrobulbar hematoma or bony impingement on the optic nerve. Even a small segment of fractured bone can result in injury to the optic nerve.

Globe injury must be also excluded when evaluating the orbits and is best accomplished by evaluating each component separately. The anterior chamber is primarily assessed for volume. Decreased volume indicates corneal laceration or anterior displacement of the lens. An increase in chamber volume suggests posterior chamber rupture. The lens position is compared with the other side to assess for dislocation (Fig. 16). The posterior chamber is primarily assessed for hemorrhage (Fig. 17). Retinal detachment can occur, especially in the setting of globe rupture, and carries a typical V-shaped configuration of subretinal fluid as seen on cross-sectional imaging. Finally, the orbit should be inspected for foreign bodies, keeping in mind that nonmetallic items, such as wood, may mimic air on CT (Fig. 18). Any concerning finding should prompt immediate ophthalmologic examination.

Fractures of the zygoma and zygomatic-maxillary complex

The zygoma is an integral part of the buttress system and articulates with 4 facial bones: the maxilla, temporal bone, sphenoid bone, and frontal bone. It provides support to the orbital contents comprising the lateral and inferior orbit. It also has cosmetic significance, comprising the malar eminence, which is the most prominent feature of the lateral midface.

Zygomatic maxillary complex (ZMC) fractures (Figs. 19 and 20) are the second most common facial fracture and result from direct blows to the malar eminence.[31] This fracture pattern crosses both the lateral buttress and the horizontally oriented inferior orbital rim buttress involving all 4 sites of articulation. Specifically, the fracture line can involve the zygomaticomaxillary, zygomaticotemporal, frontozygomatic, and zygomaticosphenoid sutures. It is important to assess all of these components when a ZMC fracture is suspected, and it is more helpful to the surgeon to classify the fracture pattern as opposed to simply naming the fractures present. Because of the 3-dimensional complexity of the fracture, reduction of the 2 buttresses can potentially leave rotational misalignment of the zygomaticosphenoid suture. If the zygomaticosphenoid fracture is not adequately reduced before addressing the remaining fractures, the facial width will be increased and the cheek will be underprojected.

Fractures of the zygoma do not always involve all 4 suture lines. The zygomatic arch is the most commonly disrupted component of the zygoma. Arch fractures occur from direct lateral force resulting in 2 distinct fracture fragments that are usually displaced medially and inferiorly. These fracture fragments can cause impingement of the temporalis muscle or coronoid process of the mandible and may impact dental occlusion.

Midface fractures

Midface fractures tend to occur along predictable locations, which correspond to relatively weak areas in the craniofacial skeleton. These classic fracture patterns were first described by René Le Fort and were based on his experiments with cadaveric skulls.[32–34] Le Fort described 3 distinct patterns: (I) palatofacial disjunction, (II) midfacial separation, and (III) craniofacial disjunction (Fig. 21). Although the patterns of these fractures differ, it is important to remember that fractures of the pterygoid processes are a necessary component of all 3 Le Fort subtypes.[35] These patterns were based on low-velocity impacts as seen in fistfights and sporting events. As the mode of injury in the modern world is predominantly high velocity secondary to vehicular collisions, the fracture patterns in these scenarios do not always conform to these classic patterns. When communicating to the surgeon, it is helpful when possible to classify a fracture pattern in addition to identifying individual fractures, although it is not always possible.

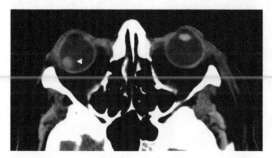

Fig. 16. A 65-year-old man involved in a motor vehicle accident as a restrained driver. Axial noncontrast orbit CT image shows dislocation of the right lens into the vitreous (*white arrowhead*).

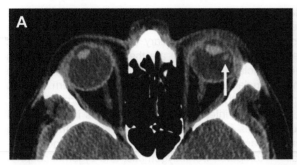
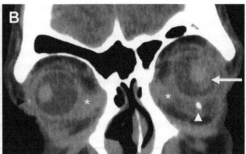

Fig. 17. A 47-year-old man presented to the emergency department after injuring his globes when he was hit with glass. Axial (*A*) and coronal (*B*) noncontrast orbit CT images show small radiopaque foreign bodies at the inferior margin of the left globe (*white arrowhead in B*) and anterior lateral margin of the right globe (*black arrowhead in B*). There is mild periorbital and soft tissue swelling/hemorrhage, left greater than right (*asterisks in B*). The left anterior chamber and vitreous contain small areas of high density, representing intraocular hemorrhage (*arrow in A, B*). Note the disconjugate gaze, concerning for extraocular musculature impairment.

Palatofacial disjunction, otherwise referred to as Le Fort I, is characterized by fracture of the anterolateral margin of the pyriform aperture immediately superior to the maxillary alveolar process (**Fig. 22**). The fracture lines extend posteriorly through the maxillary sinuses and pterygoid plates. This fracture pattern is best seen on coronal imaging. Clinically, the patient will have a mobile palate.

In midfacial separation, or Le Fort II pattern fractures, the maxilla is separated from the rest of the craniofacial skeleton. A fracture through the inferior orbital rim and floor is the unique characteristic of this fracture. The fracture continues through the nasion involving the lacrimal bone, medial orbital wall, anterolateral maxillary wall and pterygoid plates. The midface, which includes the palate, maxilla, and nose, is mobile on examination.

Le Fort III fractures, otherwise referred to as craniofacial disjunction, result in complete separation of the face from the cranium. Fracture of the lateral orbital rim and zygomatic arch is the characteristic finding of this fracture pattern. In Le Fort III fractures, the fracture line extends through the nasoethmoid complex, crosses horizontally through the medial and lateral orbital walls, traverses the pterygoid plates, and involves the zygomatic arch. The face will be completely mobile relative to the cranial vault on examination.

Although characterizing fractures using the Le Fort classification is helpful for surgical planning, it should be noted that modern day motor vehicle accidents and facial smash injuries result in a more complex pattern of trauma as compared with initial experiments by René Le Fort. Most midface fractures after motor vehicle accidents do not follow a simple Le Fort pattern; it is more common to see a combination of Le Fort fractures with additional involvement of the palate, medial maxillary arch, and dentoalveolar structures (**Fig. 23**). Most Le Fort patterns will have imperfect characteristics, and the radiologist should be careful to

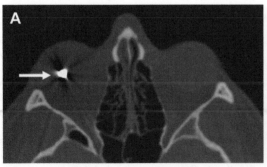
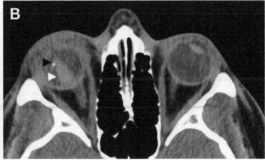

Fig. 18. A 52-year-old woman involved in a motor vehicle accident as a restrained driver, ejected through the windshield. Axial noncontrast orbit CT images show a radiopaque foreign body at the inferior margin of the right globe (*arrow in A*) and within the right vitreous (*black arrowhead in B*). The vitreous contains a wedge-shaped area of high density, representing intraocular hemorrhage (*white arrowhead in B*).

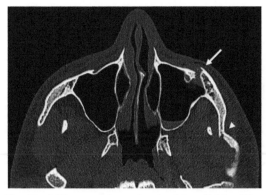

Fig. 19. A 33-year-old man involved in a fight, with a direct low-energy impact on the left zygomatic arch. Axial noncontrast facial CT image shows fracture and depression of the left zygomatic arch (*arrowhead*), with a second fracture involving the left ZMC (*arrow*).

describe in detail the fractures observed rather than simply noting a pattern. It is not uncommon to have a combined and separate pattern of Le Fort fractures on either side of the face.

Mandibular fractures
Mandibular fractures (**Fig. 24**) are frequently associated with severe midface injuries, especially Le Fort fractures. The fracture lines typically follow the long axis of the teeth, and any fracture involving dentoalveolar structures should be considered open. Given its ringlike shape, fractures of the mandible are usually accompanied by a second fracture or temporomandibular joint (TMJ) dislocation. When multiple fractures are present, one fracture approximates the site of impact and the other approximates the site of force distribution (**Fig. 25**). The latter site is

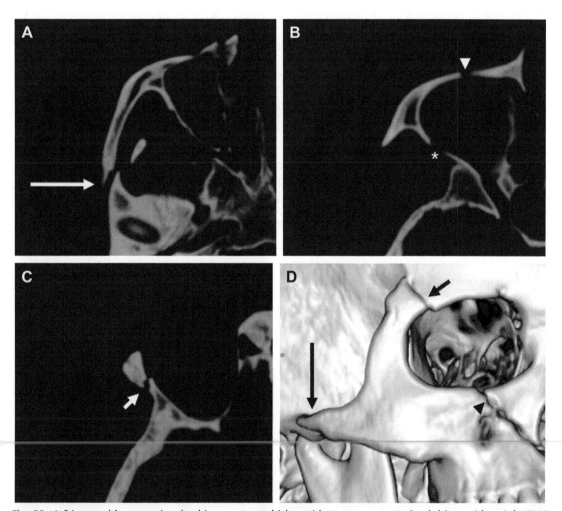

Fig. 20. A 34-year-old woman involved in a motor vehicle accident as an unrestrained driver with a right ZMC fracture. Axial noncontrast facial CT images (*A–C*) show fractures of the zygomatic arch (*long arrow*), inferior orbital rim (*arrowhead*), zygomaticosphenoid fissure (*asterisk*), and lateral orbital rim and wall (*short arrow*). 3D volume rendering of the right face (*D*) better illustrates the complexity of the fracture; again seen are fractures of the of the zygomatic arch (*long black arrow*), inferior orbital rim (*black arrowhead*), and lateral orbital rim and wall (*black short arrow*).

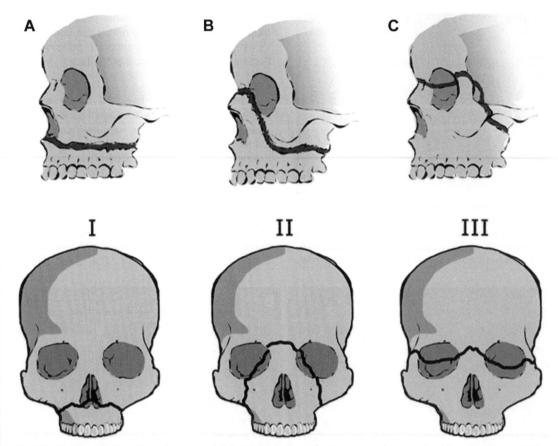

Fig. 21. Classic Le Fort pattern fractures. (*A*) Le Fort I pattern fractures are characterized by extension into the piriform aperture and palatal disjunction. (*B*) Le Fort II pattern fractures extend across the nasion and involve the inferior orbital rim. The palate and maxilla will be a mobile unit on examination. (*C*) Le Fort III fractures are characterized by fracture of the lateral orbital rim and zygomatic arch. The pterygoid plates must be fractured to be characterized a Le Fort pattern fracture.

typically the condylar neck. Condylar fracture fragments will usually displace medially and anteriorly secondary to the force of traction by the lateral pterygoid muscle, resulting in an empty glenoid fossa. Fractures through the mandibular canal may result in V3 hypoesthesia. Less commonly, bilateral TMJ dislocations can occur without fracture.

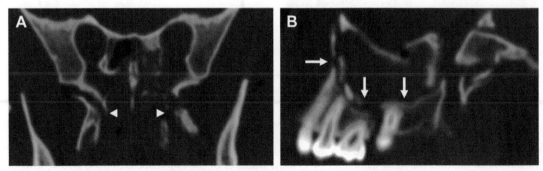

Fig. 22. A 27-year-old woman involved in a motor vehicle accident as an unrestrained driver. Le Fort I fracture. Coronal (*A*) and sagittal (*B*) noncontrast facial CT images show fractures of the bilateral pterygoid processes (*white arrowheads*), and anterolateral margins of nasal fossa above the maxillary alveolar ridge (*white arrows*).

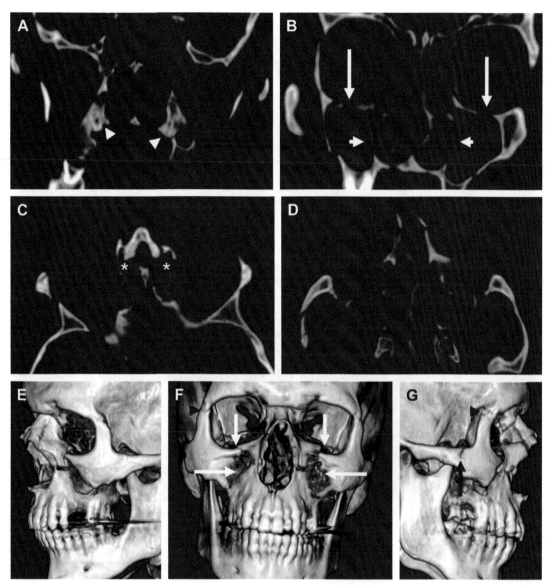

Fig. 23. A 34-year-old woman involved in a motor vehicle accident as a restrained driver. Combined Le Fort II fracture on the left and Le Fort II and III fractures on the right. Coronal noncontrast facial CT images (*A, B*) show fractures of the bilateral pterygoid processes (*white arrowheads*) and bilateral inferior orbital rims (*long white arrows*). As expected in Le Fort II fractures, the anterolateral margins of the nasal fossae are intact (*short white arrows*), thus excluding Le Fort I fracture. Axial noncontrast facial CT images (*C, D*) show fractures of the anterior portion of the medial orbital walls (*asterisks*). On the left there is also fracture of the orbital lateral rim (*black arrowhead*) and zygomatic arch (*black arrow*), features of Le Fort III fracture. 3D volume-rendered images in frontal and lateral projections (*E–G*) illustrate the previously mentioned findings (fracture of the inferior orbital rims, *white arrows* in *F*; fracture of the right zygomatic arch, *black arrow* in *G* fracture of the right orbital lateral rim *black arrowhead* in *G*).

Although many centers may screen for suspected mandible fractures with an orthopantomogram, fractures involving the condyle or ascending ramus may be missed. CT imaging is significantly more sensitive, and thus preferred, especially in the setting of high-velocity trauma where other facial fractures may be present.[36,37]

Temporal bone fractures

Temporal bone fractures have been traditionally divided into longitudinal and transverse fractures (**Fig. 26**).[38] Longitudinal fractures run parallel to the long axis of the petrous ridge and are more common than transverse fractures, representing 80% of all temporal bone fractures.[39]

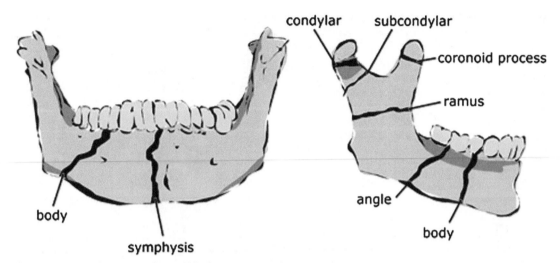

Fig. 24. Common locations of mandible fractures according to anatomic subsites. Fracture lines typically follow the long axis of the teeth. Restoring prior dental occlusion is the focal point of both open and closed treatment.

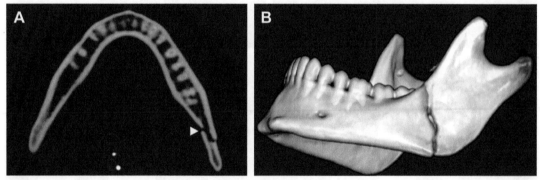

Fig. 25. A 25-year-old man involved in a fight, with direct impact to the left mandible. Axial (*A*) and 3D volume-rendered (*B*) noncontrast facial CT images show minimally displaced fracture of the left angle of the mandible (*arrowhead in A*).

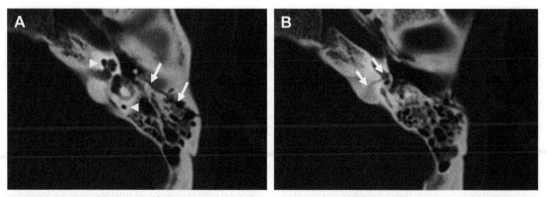

Fig. 26. A 30-year-old man who fell and struck his left ear against a hard object. Axial noncontrast temporal bone CT images (*A, B*) show nondisplaced complex fracture of the left temporal bone including both longitudinal and transverse fractures extending through the left mastoid (*arrows in A*) and the left inner ear structures (*arrows in B*). Note associated left pneumolabyrinth involving the cochlea and the posterior semicircular canal (*arrowheads*).

Although longitudinal fractures more frequently involve the internal auditory canal, damage to the otic capsule is uncommon. Conductive hearing loss is more common than sensorineural, occurring secondary to ossicular dislocation or disruption of the incudostapedial joint. Facial nerve injury is much less common (~20%) compared with transverse fractures and is usually delayed.

Transverse fractures run perpendicular to the longitudinal axis of the petrous ridge and represent the remaining 20% of temporal bone fractures. Sensorineural hearing loss is more common in transverse fractures as a result of injury to the otic capsule or cochlear nerve. Facial nerve injury occurs in 50% of transverse fractures, with immediate onset of facial paralysis reflecting either nerve compression or transection.[40] Delayed onset of facial paralysis may also occur secondary to edema or intracranial hematoma. A facial nerve hematoma may be identified as hyperintense T1 signal along the damaged nerve segment with enhancement on post-contrast T1-weighted images.[41] Facial nerve injury is the most significant finding in regard to surgical intervention, with immediate onset of complete paralysis generally indicating exploration. Delayed onset of complete paralysis may require exploration and decompression depending on the degree of nerve degeneration in the first 72 hours. Incomplete paralysis/paresis may be managed conservatively.

More recently, a new classification system has been proposed distinguishing fractures by whether they violate the otic capsule.[42] This system has been shown to be a superior predictor of clinical outcome, with otic capsule violating fractures showing significantly increased rates of facial nerve injury, CSF otorrhea, and sensorineural hearing loss. Fractures involving the otic capsule require significant force and are thus associated with more serious injury, not only to the structures housed, but the remaining craniofacial skeleton.

SUMMARY

The craniofacial skeleton and the associated viscera and soft tissue encompass a range of systems, all serviced by different medical and surgical specialists. Patients with traumatic injuries involving craniofacial anatomy will often require multidisciplinary management, and prioritizing their multiple problems is critical to providing efficient and effective care. Radiologists who are familiar with some of the chief concerns of the surgeons that manage this anatomically diverse region can help expedite the decision-making process by keeping some of these concerns in mind when they report their findings.

ACKNOWLEDGMENTS

The authors would like to thank Philip J. Cohen for creating the graphics used in **Figs. 3, 8, 21, and 24**.

REFERENCES

1. Haydel MJ, Preston CA, Mills TJ, et al. Indications for computed tomography in patients with minor head injury. N Engl J Med 2000;343(2):100–5. http://dx.doi.org/10.1056/NEJM200007133430204.
2. Stiell IG, Lesiuk H, Wells GA, et al. Canadian CT head rule study for patients with minor head injury: methodology for phase II (validation and economic analysis). Ann Emerg Med 2001;38(3):317–22. http://dx.doi.org/10.1067/mem.2001.116795.
3. Stiell IG, Wells GA, Vandemheen K, et al. The Canadian CT Head Rule for patients with minor head injury. Lancet 2001;357(9266):1391–6.
4. Stiell IG, Lesiuk H, Wells GA, et al. The Canadian CT head rule study for patients with minor head injury: rationale, objectives, and methodology for phase I (derivation). Ann Emerg Med 2001;38(2):160–9. http://dx.doi.org/10.1067/mem.2001.116796.
5. Vertinsky AT, Schwartz NE, Fischbein NJ, et al. comparison of multidetector CT angiography and MR imaging of cervical artery dissection. AJNR Am J Neuroradiol 2008;29(9):1753–60. http://dx.doi.org/10.3174/ajnr.A1189.
6. Gean AD, Fischbein NJ. Head trauma. Neuroimaging Clin N Am 2010;20(4):527–56. http://dx.doi.org/10.1016/j.nic.2010.08.001.
7. Meaney DF, Olvey SE, Gennarelli TA. Biomechanical basis of traumatic brain injury. In: Winn HR, editor. Youmans neurological surgery, vol. 4, 6th edition. Philadelphia: Elsevier Health Sciences; 2011. p. 3277–87.
8. Chestnut R, Ghajar J, Maas A, et al. The Brain Trauma Foundation. The American Association of Neurological Surgeons. The Joint Section on Neurotrauma and Critical Care. Computed tomography scan features. J Neurotrauma 2000;17(6–7):597–627.
9. Bullock MR, Chesnut R, Ghajar J, et al. Surgical management of acute epidural hematomas. Neurosurgery 2006;58(Suppl 3):S7–15 [discussion: Si–iv].
10. Bullock MR, Chesnut R, Ghajar J, et al. Surgical management of acute subdural hematomas. Neurosurgery 2006;58(Suppl 3):S16–24 [discussion: Si–iv].
11. Bullock MR, Chesnut R, Ghajar J, et al. Surgical management of traumatic parenchymal lesions. Neurosurgery 2006;58(Suppl 3):S25–46. http://dx.doi.org/10.1227/01.NEU.0000210365.36914.E3 [discussion: Si–iv].
12. Bullock MR, Chesnut R, Ghajar J, et al. Surgical management of posterior fossa mass lesions. Neurosurgery 2006;58(Suppl 3):S47–55. http://dx.doi.org/10.1227/01.NEU.0000210366.36914.38 [discussion: Si–iv].

13. Kothari RU, Brott T, Broderick JP, et al. The ABCs of measuring intracerebral hemorrhage volumes. Stroke 1996;27(8):1304–5.

14. Engelter ST, Brandt T, Debette S, et al. Antiplatelets versus anticoagulation in cervical artery dissection. Stroke 2007;38(9):2605–11. http://dx.doi.org/10.1161/STROKEAHA.107.489666.

15. Sarikaya H, da Costa BR, Baumgartner RW, et al. Antiplatelets versus anticoagulants for the treatment of cervical artery dissection: Bayesian meta-analysis. PLoS One 2013;8(9):e72697. http://dx.doi.org/10.1371/journal.pone.0072697.s004.

16. Phatouros CC, Higashida RT, Malek AM, et al. Endovascular treatment of noncarotid extracranial cerebrovascular disease. Neurosurg Clin N Am 2000;11(2):331–50.

17. Barrow DL, Spector RH, Braun IF, et al. Classification and treatment of spontaneous carotid-cavernous sinus fistulas. J Neurosurg 1985;62(2):248–56. http://dx.doi.org/10.3171/jns.1985.62.2.0248.

18. Strong EB, Pahlavan N, Saito D. Frontal sinus fractures: a 28-year retrospective review. Otolaryngol Head Neck Surg 2006;135(5):774–9. http://dx.doi.org/10.1016/j.otohns.2006.03.043.

19. Gelesko S, Markiewicz MR, Bell RB. Responsible and prudent imaging in the diagnosis and management of facial fractures. Oral Maxillofac Surg Clin North Am 2013;25(4):545–60. http://dx.doi.org/10.1016/j.coms.2013.07.001.

20. Rohrich RJ, Hollier LH. Management of frontal sinus fractures. Changing concepts. Clin Plast Surg 1992;19(1):219–32.

21. Fattahi T, Steinberg B, Fernandes R, et al. Repair of nasal complex fractures and the need for secondary septo-rhinoplasty. J Oral Maxillofac Surg 2006;64(12):1785–9. http://dx.doi.org/10.1016/j.joms.2006.03.053.

22. DeFatta RJ, Ducic Y, Adelson RT, et al. Comparison of closed reduction alone versus primary open repair of acute nasoseptal fractures. J Otolaryngol Head Neck Surg 2008;37(4):502–6.

23. Murray JA, Maran AG. The treatment of nasal injuries by manipulation. J Laryngol Otol 1980;94(12):1405–10.

24. Sargent LA. Nasoethmoid orbital fractures: diagnosis and treatment. Plast Reconstr Surg 2007;120(7 Suppl 2):16S–31S. http://dx.doi.org/10.1097/01.prs.0000260731.01178.18.

25. Rosenbloom L, Delman BN, Som PM. Facial Fractures. In: Som PM, Curtin HD, editors. Head and neck imaging. 5th edition. St Louis (MO): Mosby, Inc., an affiliate of Elsevier Inc; 2011. p. 491–524.

26. Matic DB, Tse R, Banerjee A, et al. Rounding of the inferior rectus muscle as a predictor of enophthalmos in orbital floor fractures. J Craniofac Surg 2007;18(1):127–32. http://dx.doi.org/10.1097/SCS.0b013e31802ccdc8.

27. Belli E, Matteini C, Mazzone N. Evolution in diagnosis and repairing of orbital medial wall fractures. J Craniofac Surg 2009;20(1):191–3. http://dx.doi.org/10.1097/SCS.0b013e318191ceaa.

28. Cook T. Ocular and periocular injuries from orbital fractures. J Am Coll Surg 2002;195(6):831–4.

29. Ioannides C, Treffers W, Rutten M, et al. Ocular injuries associated with fractures involving the orbit. J Craniomaxillofac Surg 1988;16(4):157–9.

30. Cullen GC, Luce CM, Shannon GM. Blindness following blowout orbital fractures. Ophthalmic Surg 1977;8(1):60–2.

31. Ochs MW. Fractures of the upper facial and midfacial skeleton. In: Myers EN, Carrau RL, editors. Operative otolaryngology: head and neck surgery, vol. 1, 2nd edition. Philadelphia: Saunders Elsevier; 2008. p. 905–33.

32. Le Fort R. Etude experimentale sur les fractures de la machoire superieure. Revue de Chirurgie de Paris 1901;23:208–27,. 360–79, 479–507.

33. Tessier P. The classic reprint: experimental study of fractures of the upper jaw. 3. René Le Fort, M.D., Lille, France. Plast Reconstr Surg 1972;50:600–7.

34. Tessier P. The classic reprint. Experimental study of fractures of the upper jaw. I and II. René Le Fort, M.D. Plast Reconstr Surg 1972;50:497–506. contd.

35. McRae M, Frodel J. Midface fractures. Facial Plast Surg 2000;16(2):107–13. http://dx.doi.org/10.1055/s-2000-12572.

36. Wilson IF, Lokeh A, Benjamin CI, et al. Prospective comparison of panoramic tomography (zonography) and helical computed tomography in the diagnosis and operative management of mandibular fractures. Plast Reconstr Surg 2001;107(6):1369–75.

37. Arosarena O, Ducic Y, Tollefson TT. Mandible fractures: discussion and debate. Facial Plast Surg Clin North Am 2012;20(3):347–63. http://dx.doi.org/10.1016/j.fsc.2012.05.001.

38. Ishman SL, Friedland DR. Temporal bone fractures: traditional classification and clinical relevance. Laryngoscope 2004;114(10):1734–41. http://dx.doi.org/10.1097/00005537-200410000-00011.

39. Nosan DK, Benecke JE, Murr AH. Current perspective on temporal bone trauma. Otolaryngol Head Neck Surg 1997;117(1):67–71.

40. Lambert PR, Brackmann DE. Facial paralysis in longitudinal temporal bone fractures: a review of 26 cases. Laryngoscope 1984;94(8):1022–6.

41. Swartz JD, Kang MD. Trauma to the temporal bone. In: Som PM, Curtin HD, editors. Head and neck imaging. 5th edition. St Louis (MO): Mosby, Inc., an affiliate of Elsevier Inc; 2011. p. 1183–229.

42. Little SC, Kesser BW. Radiographic classification of temporal bone fractures: clinical predictability using a new system. Arch Otolaryngol Head Neck Surg 2006;132(12):1300–4. http://dx.doi.org/10.1001/archotol.132.12.1300.

Index

Note: Page numbers of article titles are in **boldface** type.

Neuroimag Clin N Am 24 (2014) 553–555
http://dx.doi.org/10.1016/S1052-5149(14)00055-0
1052-5149/14/$ – see front matter © 2014 Elsevier Inc. All rights reserved.

Index

Note: Page numbers of article titles are in **boldface** type.

Printed and bound by CPI Group (UK) Ltd, Croydon, CR0 4YY

03/10/2024

01040381-0015